INTERMITTENT FASTING

Fast-Friendly Recipes for Optimal
Health, Weight Loss, and Results

COOKBOOK

NICOLE POIRIER

Founder of MindBodyKeto.com

FAIR WINDS

Inspiring | Educating | Creating | Entertaining

Brimming with creative inspiration, how-to projects, and useful information to enrich your everyday life, Quarto Knows is a favorite destination for those pursuing their interests and passions. Visit our site and dig deeper with our books into your area of interest: Quarto Creates, Quarto Cooks, Quarto Homes, Quarto Lives, Quarto Drives, Quarto Explores, Quarto Gifts, or Quarto Kids.

First Published in 2020 by Fair Winds Press, an imprint of The Quarto Group, 100 Cummings Center, Suite 265-D, Beverly, MA 01915, USA. T (978) 282-9590 F (978) 283-2742 QuartoKnows.com

Fair Winds Press titles are also available at discount for retail, wholesale, promotional, and bulk purchase. For details, contact the Special Sales Manager by email at specialsales@quarto.com
or by mail at The Quarto Group, Attn: Special Sales Manager, 100 Cummings Center, Suite 265-D, Beverly, MA 01915, USA.

24 23 22 21 20   1 2 3 4 5

ISBN: 978-1-59233-9594

Digital edition published in 2020
eISBN: 978-1-63159-887-6

Library of Congress Cataloging-in-Publication Data
Names: Poirier, Nicole, author.
Title: The intermittent fasting cookbook : fast-friendly recipes for optimal health, weight loss, and results / Nicole Poirier.
Description: Beverly : Fair Winds Press, 2020. | Includes bibliographical references and index.
Identifiers: LCCN 2020010690 (print) | LCCN 2020010691 (ebook) | ISBN 9781592339594 (trade paperback) |
   ISBN 9781631598876 (ebook)
Subjects: LCSH: Reducing diets--Recipes. | Intermittent fasting. | Intermittent fasting--Recipes. | Low-calorie diet--Recipes.
Classification: LCC RM222.2 .P5884 2020 (print) | LCC RM222.2 (ebook) | DDC 641.5/63--dc23
LC record available at https://lccn.loc.gov/2020010690
LC ebook record available at https://lccn.loc.gov/2020010691

Design: Kathie Alexander
Cover Images: Alison Bickel Photography
Page Layout: Kathie Alexander
Photography: Alison Bickel Photography
   Additional photography and Illustration: Shutterstock on pages 9, 11, 13, 21, 30, 37, 52, 54 and 57.

Printed in Canada

The information in this book is for educational purposes only. It is not intended to replace the advice of a physician or medical practitioner. Please see your health-care provider before beginning any new health program.

This book is dedicated
in loving memory of my mother,
Jeanne Marie Poirier.
If only we knew then what we know now,
this might not just be in memory.

Contents

Introduction

Our lives often revolve around feasting. We eat to celebrate, and we eat to soothe. We eat to nourish, and we eat because food tastes good. We eat, we eat, and we eat!

Although eating should be enjoyable, it is all too often stressful for many people. Are we eating enough? Are we eating too much? Are we eating the right things? What diet am I supposed to follow? The questions are endless and time consuming. As obesity rates skyrocket around the world, despite nine-thousand different gurus telling us what we should and shouldn't put into our pie holes, the questions (and pounds) continue to multiply. It's gotten to the point where every mealtime is a measurement of self-worth and that, my friends, is the opposite of healthy.

I have worked as a chef with a focus on nutritional healing for the past seventeen years. In conjunction with doctor-provided advice and as much research and testing as I can do myself, my goal has been to educate and assist my clients in finding the best way to nourish and heal their bodies one meal at a time. Over the past few years, regardless of individual dietary requirements, my most common recommendation has been less about *what* to eat and more about *when* to eat—which brings us to intermittent fasting (IF).

Intermittent fasting is basically a time-influenced pattern of eating. Your day is broken into a "fasting period" during which you consume no calories, and a "feasting window" during which you do consume calories. The fasting period gives your body a chance to rest, digest, heal, and transform the calories you have already consumed (and possibly even are storing as fat) into the energy you need to fuel your life. The feasting window provides an opportunity to restock the cellular "shelves" with the vitamins, minerals, and nutrients you need, as well as socialize and commune with friends, family, and strangers. IF is simply about intentionally timing when you eat and when you don't and making sure that you get enough hydration to support your body through both phases!

The importance of drinking water cannot be emphasized enough. Of all of the nutrients the body requires, water is the *most* important as our bodies are made up of 60 percent water and it is a necessary component of several critical biological processes. Even a small deficit can cause significant negative side effects, ranging from brain fog and cognitive impairment at just a 1 percent deficit to fatigue, irritability, headaches, and general malaise as it approaches a 4 percent deficit.

As fasting causes us to release much of the body's extra stored water by helping us break down our glycogen and release inflammation-associated edema, we need to drink more water to keep our systems in balance. A general rule of thumb is to consume at least half of your weight in ounces of water each day. Drinking enough water will support your body, and it will help with reducing hunger, too! (Particularly if you drink carbonated water during a hunger pang!)

Even though IF seems like a relatively minor tweak of an age-old practice, reports of the health benefits of IF are pouring in from all over the place.

- Fitness-minded communities hail IF as a means to increase leanness, elevate growth hormones, and speed muscle recovery (especially when combined with well-timed workout and feasting window combinations).

- Biohackers, always on the hunt to cultivate the body's optimal performance, are working with IF to change their own epigenetics (i.e., alterable gene expression) in an effort to promote longevity and prevent future disease.

- Medical professionals are incorporating IF as a means of treating diabetes, metabolic syndrome, and PCOS; lowering insulin and blood sugar; reducing blood pressure; and soothing chronic inflammation, the harbinger of advancing disease.

A 2018 peer-reviewed medical study illustrated an increase in the effectiveness in chemotherapy for certain cancer patients when they fasted prior to treatment. From a weight-loss perspective, IF is helping people successfully lose weight and also get a psychological and physiological handle on eating that many were never able to find before.

The list goes on, and that is what brings me to write this book—for *you*, wherever you are in your health journey. Now is the right time for an easy-to-read, how-to guide to demystify this seemingly "magical" yet actually very approachable practice and implement it into your life. I start with a complete overview of fasting and its many benefits, move on to explore different methods to find the one that is right for you, explain how to get started and stay on track, and finally provide you with a whole bunch of delicious, superfood-based, anti-inflammatory, ultra-nutrient-dense recipes that will inspire and nourish you at the same time.

I hope you're as excited about reading this as I am about sharing it. IF has changed the lives of many of my clients and friends, from more than one pretty-fit bride-to-be looking to get into her best shape for the wedding to multiple elderly male clients seeking to correct their blood sugar levels and stave off diabetes medications despite existing renal issues and/or congestive heart failure. (IF was undertaken with their fully informed doctors' consent and regular medical supervision.)

In my personal experience, intermittent fasting has helped me bust through a years-long weight loss plateau as well as finally get in touch with my own hunger signals. This is quite a feat because being a chef means that my entire *workday* (not just my social life, as is the case for most people) is centered on procuring, preparing, tasting, and serving food! It's been a delicious life so far, but before incorporating IF into my life I never felt this radiant. Never before did I know that feeling great and in control could be so easy, so flexible, and so forgiving.

Disclaimer

Before we go any further, I want to take a moment to say that even though I have worked in conjunction with multiple medical and nutrition professionals in the course of helping my clients, I am not a medical professional myself.

This book is not intended to be used as a substitute for medical advice. It is an educational guide only and any information in it is not to be used to diagnose and/or treat any medical condition. If you are facing a medical condition or suspect that you may be, I encourage you to seek medical advice from a qualified professional and discuss how this eating pattern may or may not have a place in combination with your existing treatment.

1

Fasting

Fasting. It's the word on everybody's lips at the moment—at the gym, the coffee shop, the school drop-off lane, and the tech company cafeteria. In the past, the word evoked ideas of deprivation and religious customs, but now it triggers thoughts of joy, productivity, healing, and almost limitless possibilities.

Fasting, particularly the carefully considered intermittent fasting (IF) balanced with highly nutritive feasting covered in this book, is being hailed as a panacea, a cure-all of sorts, with fresh success stories and anecdotes coming out regularly across mainstream media and social media outlets.

We are discussing IF like it's new, and some even deign to refer to it as a fad diet, but fasting has a long history as a spiritual, religious, and yes, health practice. Read on to learn about the basics and the health benefits of this age-old practice.

CHAPTER ONE

The Basics and Benefits of Intermittent Fasting

The term "intermittent fasting" refers to caloric reduction or restriction during previously specified time intervals. It can serve as an umbrella term for various fasting diet plans, but this definition is misleading. "Diet" tends to refer to *what* you eat, but intermittent fasting is all about *when* you eat, and just a little more focused on when you don't.

Most often people are referring to time-restricted eating (TRE) when they speak of intermittent fasting, though it does technically include alternate patterns of caloric restriction (detailed in the next chapter). TRE, or time-restricted feeding as some refer to it, consists of limiting food intake to a very specific window and abstaining from all food consumption outside of that window.

The most popular format, and the one that actor Hugh Jackman famously gives credit to for his ripped physique, is the 16:8 pattern, where nothing is consumed for 16 hours in a row before giving yourself 8 hours to enjoy your calories for the day. There is no hard rule about how long you must fast for, though it is generally accepted that 12 hours is the minimum to trigger any health benefits.

Whatever method you choose, IF is a schedule, designed by you and customized to your needs, to confidently gain control over your relationships with food, your body, and your mind. It is a health-seeking lifestyle that can free you from food obsessions and addictions, and it can enhance your health and energy levels in countless ways.

Why Does IF Make Physiological Sense?

If you've had any exposure to popular diet culture over the past thirty or so years, you've heard the advice to keep your metabolism "stoked" by eating five to six small meals per day. Sure, it *sounds* great—who wouldn't want to eat more to burn more calories? If the proof is in the (frequently eaten) pudding, then why have obesity and diabetes rates continued to steadily and sharply rise as we as a society eat more, and more often, in an attempt to become healthier?

The reason behind this is primarily hormonal and involves insulin and leptin, the so-called "satiety hormone." Leptin sends signals between your brain and cells, telling the body when its energy needs are satisfied. A steady stream of fuel in the form of food-based calories triggers the production of insulin. When your body constantly produces insulin, however, your sensitivity to leptin decreases, which tells your brain you're starving when really you are eating much more than you need.

Leptin is created in adipose, or fatty, tissue, so you might think that the more leptin your body produces, the less hungry you will be. However, the opposite happens when too much leptin is produced. The body gets overwhelmed and starts to believe that there must be an error, leading the brain to start ignoring the signals. This is commonly known as leptin resistance, the opposite of leptin sensitivity.

If the body is leptin resistant, it increases the chances of overfeeding and weight gain. Intermittent fasting helps retrain the brain and cells to recognize the signaling once again, increasing leptin sensitivity. When it comes to weight loss, studies show you actually need to lower both insulin *and* leptin to burn fat, and the only non-medicine method to do that is to take a break from eating.

That said, IF is not all about weight. It provides a rest-and-recovery opportunity for your body, that magical machine that breathes, pumps blood, and runs a zillion other life-giving processes that you don't even have to think about.

I am a chef who thinks of life in general in relation to beautiful meals and ingredients and fasting as a way to savor what you've just enjoyed. Imagine you were at the world's top restaurant and just ate the most amazing, delicious, aesthetically pleasing multi-course meal, accompanied by the perfect libations and conversation with your favorite people. As you finish your coffee, the waiter comes out and starts serving you the *next amazing meal*. You haven't had time to let the enjoyment of the last one sink in! You need a good sleep and quite possibly a belly rub. The point is that it's the time in between meals that allows you to fully appreciate and get the most out of the one you just had.

What ARE The Benefits of IF?

As you read about the advantages of intermittent fasting, you'll find even more reasons to explore it than what led you to open this book in the first place.

- **Leads to weight loss. This is the reason many people start IF, but the non-scale benefits (NSB), such as a shrinking waistline or increase in energy, often end up being the reason people stick with it. By the very nature of eating for less time during the day (or week, depending on what kind of IF you choose to do), there is a tendency to decrease overall calories without even trying, leading to weight loss.**

- **Turns your fat *against* itself. We have two types of fat: white adipose tissue (WAT) and brown adipose tissue (BAT). WAT is the jiggly stuff we don't want that stores surplus energy and hormones. BAT burns calories to create heat and energy, and increasingly it has been shown to also increase metabolism and reduce the chances for diet-induced obesity. It has been shown to promote the browning of WAT to BAT.**

- **Reduces inflammation in the body. White blood cells called monocytes float around in our bloodstreams and are testable markers for inflammation. Studies show that fasting reduces not only the number of monocytes present in the blood, but also just how inflammatory and/or harmful they are.**

10 BENEFITS OF INTERMITTENT FASTING

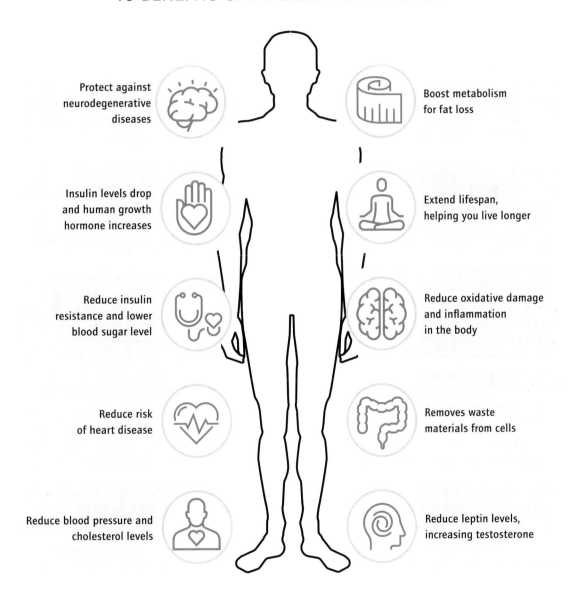

Protect against neurodegenerative diseases

Insulin levels drop and human growth hormone increases

Reduce insulin resistance and lower blood sugar level

Reduce risk of heart disease

Reduce blood pressure and cholesterol levels

Boost metabolism for fat loss

Extend lifespan, helping you live longer

Reduce oxidative damage and inflammation in the body

Removes waste materials from cells

Reduce leptin levels, increasing testosterone

- Helps improve sleep. Achieving better sleep works best when we tie our fasting schedules to our natural circadian rhythm.

- Supercharges your brain. Amazingly, IF can increase neuroplasticity, the rate at which the brain forms new neurons, the connections that bring the spark to our plugs, according to a 2005 article on meal frequency, energy intake, and health in *Annual Review of Nutrition*. This ties right into improved memory and our ability to learn and retain new information.

- Promotes longevity. Even when participants ate a less-than-ideal, inflammatory, or not particularly nutritive diet, they *still* showed increases in a much-researched gene that "promotes longevity and is involved in protective cell responses," according to a 2015 article in the journal *Rejuvenation Research.*

- Encourages cellular repair. The word of the hour here is "autophagy," which refers to when your cells eat up their own garbage as food and fuel, kind of like Doc Brown's second version of his car in *Back to the Future*! In 2016, scientist Yoshinori Ohsumi won the Nobel Prize for discovering the mechanisms of autophagy.

- Increases human growth hormone. Human growth hormone is key for muscle growth, injury recovery, body composition, and a healthy metabolism.

- Helps reduce many heart disease–related factors. These include high blood pressure, LDL (bad cholesterol), and triglyceride levels.

- May help fight cancer. IF may have positive effects on preventing cancer and also ameliorating current cancer treatment. The "may" is here because the cancer prevention studies have up until this point in time all been done on animals.

- Encourages a more communicative relationship between you and your body. Our bodies "talk" to us all the time. When we stub our toe or burn our hand on a hot pan, the messages are usually transmitted loud, clear, and fast. Messages about what does and does not make us feel good or when we are feeling hunger as opposed to boredom (raising my hand, here!) are often much subtler and can be drowned out if we aren't listening more carefully.

This list could go on and on. I have read so many studies, articles, and anecdotes in the fasting support groups I am a member of that I think the benefits are actually limitless—increased libido, freedom from binge eating, effective pain and symptom management for chronic and autoimmune conditions, increased fertility, and lower incidences of loose skin post weight loss are just a few that come to mind.

Conclusion? Fasting can be a health-seeker's dream-come-true. Now that we know the *why*, let's learn the *how!*

CHAPTER TWO

Finding the Fasting Pattern That's Right for You

Intermittent fasting is not a specific diet. Instead, it is a pattern of eating. When we define the pattern in the terms of time, we get time-restricted eating (TRE), also called time-restricted feeding. This means that a person eats all of his or her calories/meals within a specified time each day. When this will occur and for how long will vary according to the participant's own preferences and the plan they choose to follow.

Your metabolism has two basic states: fed and fasted. When we eat and are "fed," our bodies say, "Let's use as many of these calories as we can for fuel *now* and save the ones that we don't need yet for *later*. " Food is digested and then used in one of the following ways:

- converted into glucose, which is used immediately

- triggered by insulin to tuck itself into our cells for immediate use

- shuttled to the liver or muscles as glycogen for short-term storage as a fail-safe for our brains and central nervous systems

- converted to fat to use at another time

When we are "fasted," we get to tap into the "later" category. We first use up as much glycogen as we can, releasing it from the liver first as it is most easily accessible there (as opposed to the stores deeply buried in the muscles). Once glycogen stores are down, the body starts to look for more fuel options and enters a ketogenic state, which means fat (particularly triglycerides, which are the result of excess carbohydrate storage) becomes the chosen fuel source.

Important note: This transition into ketosis naturally occurs in a fasted state and does not require you to choose a ketogenic or low-carbohydrate diet. Intermittent fasting is compatible with any way of eating.

This happens all the time, to every being on the planet, whether or not they are intentionally fasting. Sleep is something of an unintentional fast, which gave rise to the word "breakfast," our earliest ingestion of calories of the day after not eating while unconscious. While we are sleeping, the body continues to metabolize calories to fuel our respiration and perspiration, regulate our body temperature and blood pressure, repair damaged cells, organs, and tissues, and strengthen our immune systems. That's a lot of work to manage! Luckily, the human body is designed for it, and we can get even better at it during both waking and sleeping hours with intentional periods of not eating.

So how do you get started tapping into this storage? How long do you have to *not* eat to start gaining the health benefits? How long *can* you fast before the benefits taper off?

It's All About the Window

This is a great time to talk about "feasting windows" or "eating windows," the chosen time periods during which we consume all our daily calories. They're referred to as windows because they open and shut and generally don't take up the whole "wall"! Typically, apart from beginner fasting, time-restricted eating windows take up less than 50 percent of the 24-hour day.

The Most Common TRE Protocols

12:12 — This indicates that you will consume all your calories within a twelve-hour period and fast for a twelve-hour period. This is the perfect regimen for someone who has not fasted before to start with.

In my experience, many people *think* they're already doing this, not realizing that coffee with cream, half and half, or milk at 6:30 a.m. or that last bite of dinner, that cookie, or that sip of wine that happened at 9:30 p.m. counts. This format requires choosing a twelve-hour period, any twelve-hour period, such as 6 a.m.–6 p.m., 7 p.m.–7a.m., 8 a.m.–8 p.m., and so on to be the time period during which you consume *all* your calories.

At the twelve-hour mark of fasting, your body fully enters a "fasted state." Food previously consumed has been used

for energy and the digestive system gets an opportunity to rest. With this major metabolic function on pause, energy can be diverted to healing processes. Human growth hormone (HGH) production begins to increase and glucagon is released to keep blood sugars balanced by signaling the conversion of stored glycogen in the liver and muscles into glucose for necessary processes.

14:10 — This is the next step up on the ladder, increasing the fasting period to fourteen hours while decreasing the "feeding window" to ten hours. An example might be having breakfast at 9 a.m. and finishing dinner no later than 7 p.m.

This time configuration allows for more cooperation with your circadian rhythm (your internal body clock that governs your sleep/wake cycles in response to light and dark) and master biological clock, a group of about 20,000 neurons located in the hypothalamus called the "suprachiasmatic nucleus" (SCN). It also still allows for a regular social life! Also, at fourteen hours, there is a pronounced and dramatic increase in HGH production. The body starts to tap into the fat stores to use for energy.

16:8 — This is currently the most read, written-about, and practiced strategy. All calories must be consumed in an eight-hour period followed by a sixteen-hour fasting period. Many early-stage intermittent fasters find it relatively easy to transition to this type of window, either skipping traditional breakfast and eating two meals between noon and 8 p.m. or starting a little earlier in the day, such as 9 a.m., and having breakfast, lunch, and possibly a pre-fast snack later in the afternoon, closing the window at 5 p.m.

This format was initially introduced and popularized by trainer Martin Berkhan, who called it the Leangains method. Leangains has been credited with the aforementioned transformation of Hugh Jackman—but simply following the time restriction does not involve the in-depth protocols or strict dietary, supplement, and workout adherence that Leangains specifies.

Eating methodology aside, we normally sleep about eight hours per night, which leaves eight additional hours of uninterrupted not-eating. With conventional wisdom and plenty of peer-reviewed studies recommending discontinuing eating a few hours before bedtime, the 16:8 method also truly accommodates our circadian rhythm, because this type of monitored calorie consumption flows with the biologically-scheduled rest periods for our internal organs as well as light-dark-assisted hormone production.

There are other huge advantages to extending the fasting window as fat-burning at this point becomes much more consistent. The sweet spot is eighteen to twenty-four hours of fasting for maximum fat-burning and autophagy, a rejuvenating process in which your body cleans up and recycles its own "junk cells" as fuel. Sixteen hours of fasting tips the human body into the fully fasted fat-burning zone.

This format is great for maintaining social connection with meals. One of the greatest challenges IF-ers face is explaining to friends, family, and coworkers why they are not eating. Not that it's anybody's business but your own, but you will receive plenty of critical comments, peer pressure, and possibly outright attempts at sabotage. Stay strong and remember, you are doing this for your health and well-being, not to make anybody else feel comfortable in *their* skin.

20:4 — You likely understand the window formats by now, and this one includes a twenty-hour fasting period followed by a four-hour feasting window. Clearly, this protocol is a more intense fasting regime. Participants may eat one large meal at some point during the window, break it up into a snack and a meal, or consume a few small snacks.

One version of this protocol is the Warrior Diet, written about and popularized by author and fitness expert Ori Hofmekler in 2001. Having served in the Israeli Special Forces, Hofmekler combined his personal experience with historical research into societies such as the Spartans and Romans to formulate what might be considered the first popular foray into promoting intermittent fasting as a sustainable way of life. This protocol does not necessarily advocate a completely calorie-free fasting window, allowing for tiny amounts of specifically recommended low-calorie foods if hunger becomes unbearable before one large, preferable whole-foods-based meal in the evening. This particular protocol also recommends a daily workout in the fasted state.

With the extension of the fasting window to twenty hours, natural creation of HGH soars. This is a great time to build muscle while also burning fat, which may be why a workout is built into the Warrior Diet protocol.

One Meal a Day (OMAD) — This format sounds simple and self-explanatory, but it depends on where you get your information! The most accepted notion is to eat only one large, nourishing, and highly caloric meal per day in a one-hour period, honoring a 23:1 fasting/feasting time frame. This extended fasting window gives the body one of the most significant fat-burning time periods while still eating daily, and it's much more difficult to overdo the calories assuming you are choosing real, whole foods as opposed to heavily processed ones. Also, once you get into the swing of things, hunger drops dramatically and the time and amount of food it takes to feel full also decline.

Author and IF advocate Gin Stephens of *Delay, Don't Deny* is not as strict as far as defining the timing window so long as the contents of that window constitute just one meal. For instance, a snack may be consumed while preparing dinner to open the OMAD window, followed by a dinner consisting of a few courses and closing out with a glass of wine and little dessert. She makes the argument for eating as if you are at a fine-dining establishment: you would not rush a multi-course meal if it were being prepared for you at a restaurant, and it is still just one meal you have there.

I appreciate this approach and follow it myself most days with my own window varying between one and four hours depending on the setting and situation. It seems to me to be the most conducive to enjoying my meals without feeling rushed and leaving enough space and awareness to recognize my body's satiety signals.

Most people who follow the OMAD schedule will harness nutritional ketosis regardless of what they eat, and that comes along with its own anti-inflammatory benefits as well as sharply increased levels of HGH and autophagy. As previously mentioned, between eighteen and twenty-four hours fasted is known as the sweet spot of fat burning, in which the greatest concentration of stored fat is mobilized to convert to energy.

Alternate Day Fasting (ADF)

Where TRE is an intermittent fasting pattern repeated every day, alternate day fasting (ADF) is one that is practiced either every other day or just a few times per week. On fasting days, calories are restricted to about 25 percent of normal or less, and on feasting days one can consume foods normally. That might sound too good to be true, but research has shown that most people only consume an extra 500 calories on their feast days, which is still a fraction of what is NOT consumed on fasting days! Of course, overconsumption of calories and binging on non-fasting days can be detrimental to weight loss efforts, if not cause weight gain; "normal" eating refers to the same level of calories you would have consumed had you not been fasting the day before.

ADF can provide the same health benefits as TRE. Followers of these protocols will still lose weight, gain the benefits of autophagy, and preserve muscle mass while shedding fat. In addition, it reduces the chances of adaptive thermogenesis (a.k.a. "starvation mode,") that traditional calorie restriction diets often trigger. Over-restricting calories over time will cause the body to want to preserve the status quo and decrease the number of calories it needs to stay the same weight and even gain weight more easily. Keeping healthy thermogenesis (the increase in heat and energy expenditure after eating due to digestion and muscles gobbling up their new fuel) is critical to weight loss and weight loss maintenance.

The biggest challenges people tend to face with ADF are calorie creep on fasting days and longer-term adherence due to social factors. That said, ADF is a safe, effective form of intermittent fasting that has helped countless practitioners around the world improve their health.

The Most Common ADF Protocols

Crescendo Method — This method of fasting for twelve to sixteen hours three days per week on nonconsecutive days has gained some press for being particularly female-friendly and is indeed an easy way to start transitioning into ADF. That said, research does not fully support the claims that women necessarily need to fast differently than men, according to top IF researcher Krista Varady, Ph.D. Still, this is a great warm-up method.

Eat Stop Eat — Fitness guru Brad Pilon created this method while doing graduate research on short-term fasting at the University of Guelph in Ontario, Canada. Eat Stop Eat requires two twenty-four-hour fasts per week and "responsible eating" the other five days. ("Responsible eating" entails planning, eating mindfully, and coping when your plan goes awry.) That means for two days per week, you might finish eating your dinner one day at 8 p.m. and not eat again until the following day at 8:01 p.m., but there *is* eating every day.

The twenty-four-hour fasts still reduce overall weekly caloric intake without putting any limitations on what you choose to consume. Eat Stop Eat also sparks nutritional ketosis, even if only for a short period, promoting that fat-burning!

The Fast Diet/5:2 — The Fast Diet was created by British journalist Michael Mosely in 2012 (updated in 2017) and the basic rules were further popularized by author and journalist Kate Harrison with her *5:2 Diet* book in 2013. Since then, there have been countless cookbooks, guides, and other publications to help consumers adhere to this easy plan.

The idea is to consume only 500 calories if you're a woman, 600 if you're a man, on two nonconsecutive days of the week and eat normally the remaining five days. On "fasting" days, people generally consume three very small meals in typical breakfast-lunch-dinner fashion or two slightly larger meals for lunch and dinner. This method requires meal planning and calorie counting, but only for two days per week.

The Every Other Day Diet/Modified Alternate Day Fasting — Krista Varady, Ph.D., a nutritionist and one of the world's top and most-published researchers on the subject of IF, designed and wrote a book about this manner of ADF. Instead of choosing two random nonconsecutive days during which to consume 500 calories, Varady recommends implementing that same version of fasting literally every other day, setting the body on a predictable 48-hour schedule. The ability to adapt to a schedule reportedly makes *this* version of ADF easier than others, according to her research.

Much like the 5:2 diet, there are no hard and fast (pun intended!) rules about what you can eat on feast days, but

Varady's research does point to ingesting higher fat foods, leading to higher levels of both satiety and weight loss.

Intuitive Fasting

Intuitive fasting is loosely defined. It basically entails skipping meals and eating when you feel like it as opposed to relying on any particular pattern, structure, or schedule. Instead, like intuitive eating in general, intuitive fasting implies that those who practice it have a high level of communication with their bodies and are able to define both what makes a body feel good and what true hunger signals are.

We have already established that fasting is not unhealthy. However, the efficacy of intuitive fasting for achieving the health-based benefits discussed earlier does not have any solid merit. It is extremely difficult to eat intuitively and clearly hear the body's communication if one is not consuming whole food ingredients. Highly processed foods are designed in laboratories to trick satiety signals and cause consumers to want more.

There is some aspect of intuitive eating involved in every form of intermittent fasting, regardless of what dietary plan one chooses to follow. Each and every protocol encourages fasters to eat until they are full, but it's the abstinence outside of the feast that delivers the decreased insulin, fat-burning, and so on.

The one situation where intuitive fasting may induce some of the typical health benefits of IF is when one is already following a very low-carbohydrate or ketogenic diet. Because these types of diets already have the body cleared of glucose, stored glycogen, and therefore insulin, skipping meals here and there may happen as a natural result of lowered hunger and result in a greater use of fat stores.

Extended Fasting

As both TRE and ADF are built to accommodate twelve- to twenty-four-hour periods of fasting, anything over that is considered an extended fast. Although the health benefits of fasting may increase the longer one fasts in general, the potential risks also increase. (To be honest, the benefits do max out at a certain point.)

DISCLAIMER: Again, I am not a medical professional, but an experienced faster, biohacker, and healing nutrition facilitator. It is my strong belief that longer fasts should not be undertaken without serious preparation (e.g., regular IF for multiple weeks and a lower carbohydrate diet), if not medical supervision, especially for those currently prescribed medication for diabetes and other chronic conditions.

That said, there are medical professionals such as fasting gurus Jason Fung, M.D., Rhonda Patrick, Ph.D., and Annette Bosworth, M.D., among others, who are serious advocates for extended fasting and incorporate 36- to 72-hour fasts into their programs and personal lives.

Practitioners use extended or prolonged fasting for a number of reasons. Sometimes it's as simple as breaking through a weight loss plateau, or stall. It could be for immune system regeneration or increased HGH production. There are plenty of worthwhile reasons to consider adding prolonged fasting into your schedule, but it is certainly something that involves preparation, and restricting calories is *not* recommended once the fasting period is over. Eating normally to satiety is preferred.

In the event that you do attempt any of the following prolonged fasting schedules, listen to your body and *stop* if you feel unwell or faint. Supplement your electrolytes and stay hydrated. Take care to break your fast with something gentle and low-glycemic, such as warm lemon water and a handful of almonds, about an hour before you feast normally. Remember that although supervised fasting for more than 72 hours is possible, basal metabolic rate starts to decrease after that amount of time—as opposed to anywhere up to three days, it increases. Longer isn't always better!

Most Frequently Discussed Extended Fasts
36-Hour Fast — The 36-hour fast involves skipping an entire day of eating. If, for instance, you finish eating dinner at 8 p.m. on a Monday, you would not eat again until 8 a.m. on Wednesday.

Fung incorporates 36-hour fasting two to three times per week for many of the severely overweight, Type 2 diabetic participants in his Intensive Dietary Management (IDM) program, citing expedited fat loss and greater success in the fight against insulin resistance. That's basically eating every other day without the 500-calorie boost of modified alternate day fasting.

These patients are under medical supervision, but having done these fasts myself, I can say that there are really no side effects apart from the occasional (and completely bearable) hunger pang. That's just ghrelin, our hunger hormone, letting us know that it's around the time we normally eat!

After 36 hours of fasting, it is said that metabolic rate actually *increases* (probably due to an increase in norepinephrine) and autophagy is raised *300 percent.*

If you want to return to a 16:8, 18:6, 20:4 schedule after your 36-hour fast, that is fine. You just need to adjust your eating window accordingly.

48-Hour Fast — Just like it sounds, a 48-hour fast requires no eating for two days. For best results, you would start this prolonged fast after finishing dinner a little earlier on, say, a Monday at 5 p.m. and finish at 5 p.m. on a Wednesday. This way, you have that time to gently open your window with a small snack such as a salad, handful of almonds, or cup of bone broth to wake your digestive system up and prepare yourself for a satisfying feast while also staying true to your circadian rhythm and finishing your feasting at least three hours before you go to sleep. By 48 hours, autophagy will have increased an additional 30 percent, but note that the law of diminishing returns remains in effect.

72-Hour Fasts — A 72-hour fast is quite an undertaking for an inexperienced faster, but relatively easy for an experienced one. Three days of not eating, much like the 48-hour fast, will require careful fast-breaking in order to keep your body happy, but the benefits may be worth the effort.

But *why* would you not eat for three days? Not for sustained weight loss—the dividends of a fast of this length come in other health improvements. Fat loss will continue, but weight may rebound when you begin to eat normally again. Autophagy and metabolic rate continue to increase

until the 72-hour mark, at which point they max out and start to decrease rapidly.

Valter Longo, Ph.D., a professor, cell biologist, biogerontologist, major fasting advocate, and author of *The Longevity Diet*, has done extensive research on the advantages of fasting in both humans and mice and proven that there are huge benefits to the immune system in fasting for three days, clearing out old immune cells, and producing new, healthy ones. His research also points to the benefits of this type of prolonged fast lasting for up to six months!

How do you do it? First of all, work up to it with a regular IF schedule and start incorporating 36- to 48-hour fasts. Once you can get through these with relative ease and know how to confidently handle bouts of hunger, you can take the next step. It is advisable to do your first 72-hour fast when you have a three-day period that doesn't require much energy and during which you can rest whenever you need. These fasts will get easier as you practice prolonged fasting more frequently, but 72-hour fasts are not required often if you are intending them as a tool for immune system and/or stem cell regeneration.

Longer Fasts (3+ Days) — There aren't many scientific studies on fasts longer than three days and almost no studies performed include zero calorie consumption. There does, however, appear to be plenty of anecdotal information on the internet. Having done an awful lot of background investigation, I found that many of the people promoting their weight loss success via prolonged fasting either disappeared from the public eye or gained their weight back.

That said, there are definitely targeted health benefits to doing longer fasts, particularly for experienced fasters. With close monitoring of blood sugar, hormone, and electrolyte levels to ensure your body is getting the support it needs, they can be and currently are used as tools for healing. Longer fasts show promise in enhancing stem cell regeneration and HGH production.

Longer fasts come with more risks than the versions of intermittent fasting previously discussed: There is greater loss of lean muscle mass per pound with longer fasts.

Reducing food intake for weeks will cause metabolism to slow. Many people who've used this method have reported gaining all their weight back, making it a pretty ineffective weight loss strategy in the long term. Approach longer fasts with care, make sure you're doing them for the right reasons, and seek professional guidance and monitoring to make sure your health stays in check. By all means, if you start feeling unwell, *stop*.

Additional Modified Fasting Techniques

Modified fasting is defined by eating very small amounts of food on fasting days while still getting the benefits of fasting. Technically, a number of the alternate day fasting methods include modified fasting with the consumption of 500 to 600 calories on fasting days. The techniques described below include calories, though restricted, on all days. The practices are consistent on consecutive days.

Fast-Mimicking Diet — Valter Longo has done some of the most clinical research on fasting in the world. Using decades' worth of research, he developed and patented this five-day, high-fat, low-calorie protocol to mimic the effects of fasting while still providing the body with adequate nutrition.

The diet has two caloric phases. On days 1 and 2, you consume 10 to 16 calories per kilogram (2.2 pounds) of body weight, with 10 percent coming from protein, 56 percent coming from fat, and 34 percent coming from carbohydrates. On days 3 through 5, you consume 7 to 11 calories per kilogram (2.2 pounds) of body weight, with 9 percent coming from protein, 44 percent from fat, and 47 percent coming from carbohydrates. If one wants to embark on a ketogenic version of this, calories stay the same but percentages change, with 25 percent of calories coming from protein, 70 percent from fat, and 5 percent from carbohydrates.

Whichever method you choose, it is designed to supply 34 to 54 percent of normal caloric intake but still replicates the cellular regeneration, fat loss, and decreased inflammation that normal fasting provides. The process is also intended to be repeated every one to six months to achieve optimal results.

You can try this plan on your own with the formulas provided above, but Longo has designed a prepackaged version called the ProLon Fasting Mimicking Diet available through a nutrition tech company called L-Nutra. If you decide to do it yourself with the formulas provided (included in Longo's original patent), it is highly recommended that you prepare and prepackage all meals in advance, especially if you are not coming from a low-carbohydrate or ketogenic diet that would already be helping to mitigate hunger.

Protein Sparing Modified Fast (PSMF) — The PSMF is a very low-calorie diet designed to help people lose weight and fat very quickly while preserving lean muscle mass, thereby protecting the resting metabolic rate. It is recommended only for extremely overweight people with a BMI over 30 if they are healthy or over 27 if they are suffering from type 2 diabetes, fatty liver disease, high cholesterol, sleep apnea, or osteoarthritis.

There are two phases to the diet:

- **The Intensive Phase: This phase is followed for up to a maximum of six months and usually constitutes less than 800 calories per day for every day this phase is followed. Patients eat 1.2 to 1.5 grams of protein per kilogram (2.2 pounds) of their goal body weight each day. Fat is limited to *only* what is contained in the lean-as-possible protein sources that are recommended and carbohydrates are limited to 20 grams per day.**

- **The Refeeding Phase: This phase lasts for two months and gradually introduces higher levels of fat and carbohydrates back in while protein is being reduced. Carbs are increased to 45 grams in the first month and 90 grams in the second month while protein is reduced by 40 grams in each of the months.**

People have lost a lot of weight practicing PSMF, with the average being 40 pounds (18 kg) in the first twelve weeks, according to one small study published in *JAMA* in 1993. However, one must remember that adherents start from obese weights in general, which usually coincides with rapid weight loss. The diet is *highly* restrictive, essentially combining a very low-calorie diet with a very low-carbohydrate diet. It is not recommended to do PSMF unsupervised by a medical professional, and weight rebound of at least 50 percent is extremely common.

Because calories are so low, micronutrient requirements are often very difficult to meet, and the only way to know if you're not getting them is via clinical testing.

If this method seems like something you'd still want to try despite its extremely restrictive long-term nature, consult with your doctor. The plan excludes alcohol and is very challenging when trying to maintain a social life in the long term.

CHAPTER THREE

Frequently Asked Questions

I bet you have a lot of questions! In this chapter, I address some of the most frequently asked questions, such as how to begin an IF, what kind of side effects may occur and how to deal with them, and when you'll start to see results. Let's start, however, with *who should avoid* fasting.

Who Should Not Fast?

Intermittent fasting is an incredible tool that can offer benefits to so many people, but it is not appropriate for everyone. People who should avoid IF include:

- Pregnant and breastfeeding women because their caloric needs are higher to provide for the growth of the baby

- Children and adolescents, who require more consistent nutrition to fuel periods of rapid growth

- People who are already underweight with a BMI of 18

- Those who have a history of eating disorders such as anorexia, bulimia, binge eating disorder, and orthorexia, which can be exacerbated by fasting periods

- People suffering from high stress and/or adrenal fatigue.

IF *enhances* the production of stress hormones including cortisol, norepineph-rine, and epinephrine (a.k.a. adrenaline). Cortisol tells the body to release glucose into the bloodstream for immediate use and stops insulin from helping to clear it. Ongoing stress and/or a dysfunctional adrenal response due to constant cortisol production can have a seriously detrimental effect on blood glucose levels, insulin resistance, and even the ability to sleep. Underlying stress and cortisol production need to be addressed before attempting IF.

People who should approach IF with caution include:

- Diabetics (type 1 or type 2) on medication would be best served by first discussing IF with their doctor to safely regulate their insulin levels. Diabetics have found relief through intermittent fasting, according to a small study by Jason Fung, M.D., but were under consistent professional medical supervision.

- Those suffering from anxiety and/or depression may experience an increase in symptoms and a decrease in mood as their blood sugar and gut flora adjust to IF. That said, in online fasting forums and groups, many people report *improvements* in symptoms after a short time, but the potential increase in symptoms should be considered.

- Women attempting to conceive. Significant caloric restriction changes the body's hormonal responses, specifically that of the stress and sex hormones, and may interfere with fertility. Alternate daily fasting is never recommended. A TRE schedule of sixteen or fewer fasting hours and adequate caloric intake could be safe but is not recommended. As always, consult with your medical provider.

How Do I Start?

This part is simple, but not necessarily easy, to follow. If you currently eat whatever you want whenever you want, any fasting method might feel like a challenge. Going from five or six small meals per day to two meals per day will be a big adjustment, but it *is* very doable. Choose which primary method—TRE or ADF—you think will best suit your lifestyle and begin with the least complicated structure for a week.

If eating consistently every day sounds right for you, for instance, begin with a 12:12 or 14:10 format and get your body used to precise feasting window "opening" and "closing" times. Think of this approach as training wheels. Once you're used to that slightly later breakfast or slightly

earlier dinner, you can experiment with shortening your window a little more until you find *your* sweet spot.

Does ADF sound more doable to you? Practice with the Crescendo Method (see page 16) before moving on to a regimen with more significant caloric restriction.

My advice while you are doing either method is to reduce refined sugars and carbohydrates and processed foods by adding more whole foods to your diet. There are no restricted foods in IF but taking steps to regulate your blood sugar will make the transition much easier.

How Long Will It Take to Adjust to a Fasting Lifestyle?

Like any new practice, making intermittent fasting a habit will take time. Most people get into the swing of things in just one or two weeks; I recommend giving it at least four weeks before asking yourself whether this lifestyle is right for you. By that time, most practitioners feel so good, they have forgotten what life *without* fasting was like!

What Are Common Side Effects When Transitioning to a Fasting Lifestyle?

During those first few weeks, you will experience common side effects, but don't be discouraged because they will subside once your body adjusts.

Hunger — No surprise here, as you're changing a major lifestyle routine that your body has become used to—when and how you eat. Your fabulous, intelligent, human machine has noted your shift in eating patterns and adapted hormonal signaling accordingly, though sometimes not at all at the same speed, as in the case of leptin and insulin resistance. Ghrelin, the hormone that tells your body when to get hungry, doesn't seem to face the same resistance—ever. So your efficient brain says "Hey, ghrelin! It's thirty minutes before our normal lunchtime—let everybody know!" Ghrelin, responsible little hunger hormone that it is, does just that. The level of ghrelin rises in the bloodstream before anticipated mealtimes.

Happily, your brain and hormonal systems can be retrained. It just takes a little time. You can help by drinking plenty of water and appetite suppressing beverages such as mineral water, black coffee, green tea, black tea, or unsweetened herbal, ginger, and cinnamon teas.

Cravings — These are usually for calorie-dense, but not nutrient-dense, foods and arise because you're attempting to avoid all the unhealthy foods, which clearly makes you want them more. Think about that person you dated in high school whom your parents couldn't stand—the more forbidden the fruit, the more tempting it is.

There is also a physical component to cravings, too, *especially* in the beginning. Excessive sugar consumption has been shown to light up the same reward centers in the brain as addictive illicit drugs and reducing consumption due to limiting the hours per day you eat may create a physical withdrawal period marked by intense cravings.

Cut yourself a little slack here and make sure you are eating to satiety when you *are* feasting and including plenty of healthy fats. If you really want something in particular, indulge in a little during your eating window. When nothing is off limits, cravings go away more quickly.

Mood Changes/Irritability — Mood changes in the early days of intermittent fasting arise from psychological and physiological causes. When your brain is switching from being glucose-fueled to being fat-adapted, the initial lowered blood sugar can create a physical response that manifests as an emotional response. Being able to anticipate this, however, makes a significant difference. Even if you weren't anticipating it, the potential moodiness and/ or irritability may pass in as few as three days.

I had a client who would get cranky if she didn't have something to eat first thing in the morning. Once I explained that IF would help her with pre-wedding body recomposition and was totally safe, her morning "hangries" disappeared (see "Why Am I Losing Inches When the Scale Isn't Moving?" on page 27). Her husband actually wrote to thank me!

You might feel a little irritable when your blood sugar first starts to drop, but recovery is swift, especially if you fill your feasts with the varied, nutrient-dense, whole foods discussed in this book. A varied diet not only supplies the body with the vitamins and minerals that it needs to feel at peak mood, it also supports a healthy gut microbiota. It is in the gut that 95 percent of the body's serotonin (also known as the happiness hormone and the one body chemical upon which most antidepressants act) is produced.

For a short-term solution, if you feel like you've put on particularly grumpy pants in your early days of IF, take a deep breath and thank yourself for the improved health you're about to experience. I like to think of it as telling the truth in advance, and while it may seem overly simple, science proves that even small, unspoken bouts of gratitude boost happiness and mood among even more health benefits.

Note: Of course, there are many more factors, hereditary and environmental, that shape your overall mood and emotional well-being. If you experience extreme and concerning mood shifts despite eating healthfully during your feasting window, please consult with a medical professional.

Headaches — Headaches are a typical occurrence when you first start to fast, or even transition to a lower-carbohydrate diet, and they're believed to be caused by a deficiency in electrolytes, particularly sodium. Combat this by adding a pinch of pink Himalayan or natural sea salt to each of your non-caloric drinks, having a glass of "sole" water (water saturated with pink Himalayan salt) in the morning, taking a shot of yummy, salty pickle brine/ pickle juice (no kidding!), dipping your fingertip into pink or sea salt and licking it a few times per day, or merely making sure your food is well-salted when you eat. When I am doing longer fasts, I have fingertip-dips throughout the day and they keep me feeling tip-top.

Digestive Issues — Bloating, which can happen as your gut flora adjust to new conditions, is usually *very* temporary. Constipation is normal because you are eating less and creating less waste! Making sure you get plenty of fibrous fruits and veggies during your feasting periods will help, as will taking a daily magnesium supplement. Heartburn usually comes from overeating or lying down too soon after eating. Be mindful of fullness cues, continue to drink that water, and try not to recline for at least 30 minutes to an hour after eating. Raising the head of your bed and sleeping on your left side can help if you are prone to nighttime heartburn. If you get a sharp attack—day or night—stirring ½ to 1 teaspoon of baking soda (sodium bicarbonate) into water will help alleviate it almost immediately while also giving you a good dose of sodium. Be aware that if you use this method, you may see water weight gains on the scale the next morning, but they are *nothing* to worry about.

Feeling Cold — This happened to me all the time when I started IF. When you fast, blood flow to your fat stores increases, drawing away from your extremities. This is because your body is mobilizing fat to your muscles so it can be used for fuel and is called "adipose blood flow." Turning on the blood flow turns on the fat-burning! So, put on another layer of clothes, and have a hot cup of tea or coffee to celebrate. Once your body adapts to fasting, this feeling will go away. If it's really bothersome, try supplementing with vitamin B1. Feeling cold *all* the time is not a typical fasting side effect and may be something to ask your medical provider about.

Altered Sleep Patterns — These are due to hormonal adaptation. Longer fasting periods increase cortisol and norepinephrine, which can make you feel extra energetic at bedtime. This state generally doesn't happen with regular, daily IF. My recommendation is to understand that this may be part of a longer fast and take advantage of the energy boost to get a little extra work done. Your sleeping patterns will go back to normal the next time you eat. If you *are* experiencing it with regular IF, it may be time to look at your sleep hygiene and caffeine intake, adjusting as necessary.

Reduced Energy — It is also normal to feel more tired during the transition period as your body moves away from being glucose-reliant. Time is the only cure for reduced energy, taking up to three weeks. If you can't get extra sleep at night or via catnaps during the day, my favorite wake-up-right-now ways are doing some kind of rapid, short-term exercise (such as ten to twenty jumping jacks or dancing to a short, upbeat song) or cold water immersion (cold plunge, cold shower, or even just submerging your arm or splashing your face with very cold

water). Trust me, you will wake up and not over-caffeinate yourself to prevent sleeping later.

Bad Breath — Also known as keto breath, this is a sign of fat burning and nutritional ketosis. When in ketosis, what your brain doesn't use is released. Not everybody gets it, and it doesn't usually last forever when or if you do. Drink more water and keep good dental hygiene.

Frequent Urination and/or Night Sweats — For every gram of glycogen, our stored glucose, that we burn, we release 4 grams of water. If you're following the fasting protocol, you've likely also upped your water intake! These factors result in more trips to the bathroom and sometimes, sweating like mad at night. It's all a normal part of the process but might be helped by supporting the liver with dandelion tea and stopping consumption of liquids by 7 p.m.

Muscle Cramps — Muscle cramps are typically a sign of not getting enough magnesium. You can supplement with caplets, magnesium powder, spray, or simply soaking in an Epsom salt bath each day for 30 minutes. The last is my favorite option—who doesn't love a warm, relaxing bath and want a reason to take one every day?

Is There a Best Time to Fast?

There isn't so much a best time to fast as there is a best time to feast, and this has to do with timing it just right to your circadian rhythm. The light-dark cycle gives your body cues when to create wake- and sleep-inducing hormones, when to prime the body for insulin production, and when to take a break. Our pancreas, which regulates insulin secretion, "goes to sleep" around 8 p.m. when sleep-inducing melatonin begins to be released and binds to pancreatic receptors.

The following graphic illustrates some of the most significant hormone-related times in a typical human circadian rhythm.

At this point, there will be less available insulin to handle

The Circadian Biological Clock, Hour by Hour

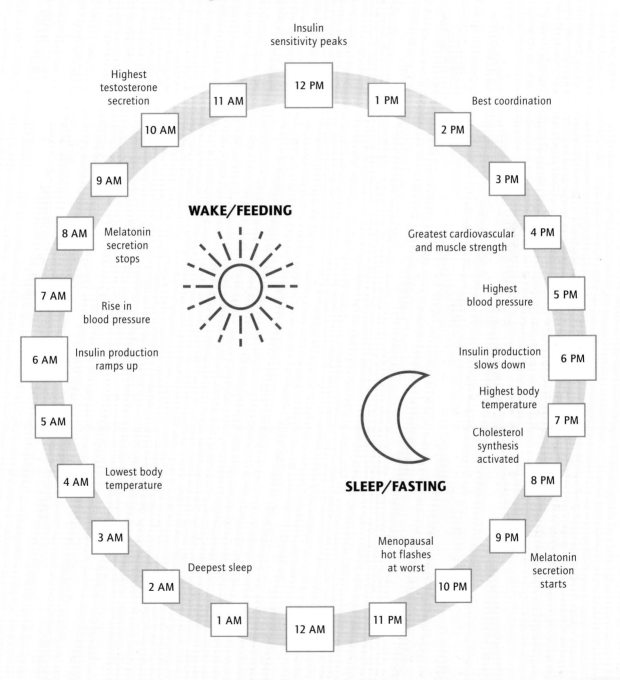

blood sugar increases resulting from consumed energy (a.k.a. food!) and *boom*—you have elevated blood sugar. Chronic exposure can lead to metabolic disorders, diabetes, and even affect your memory and concentration.

This is one of the primary reasons you see so many eating windows ending at 8 p.m. and advice telling you to stop eating a few hours before bedtime. Late-night eating leads to higher blood glucose and potentially greater insulin resistance in the long run.

Bottom line, the very least thing you can do is stop consuming calories a few hours before you go to bed for the most health benefits.

How Long Do I Need to Intermittent Fast?

There is no hard and fast rule for how long to IF. It depends entirely on your objective. Some people may use it as a tool for a few weeks to lose a small, specific amount of weight, and then revert to previous eating patterns and only use it again, or alter the schedule, to maintain the loss as needed. Others may be employing IF to try and reverse insulin resistance, balance out hormones, gain muscle, lose large amounts of weight, or trigger deeper physical healing—and these goals may take significantly more time to achieve, as in months or years.

In conversations with clients and friends who practice IF, and reflective of my own personal experience, most fall in love with the way that they feel both mentally and physically and express the intention to incorporate it into their lifestyle forever. This may or may not ring true for you, too—just remember that the key characteristic of IF is flexibility.

Can I Change My Eating Window?

Of course you can change your eating window! You are never locked into just one fasting schedule. You may have to try out different options as you get used to IF to find

what suits you best and even then, you can change hours to accommodate social functions without doing any long-term damage. In fact, your body may benefit from the occasional metabolic confusion.

The important thing to remember is that intermittent fasting is a lifestyle, not a diet. "Intermittent" means "not all the time." Feel free to be flexible. If you see yourself losing ground that you have previously gained, tighten up your commitment until you are back on track again.

Do I Need to Count Calories?

Not really. At the beginning, people tend to overeat. It might be because you feel like you're starving after fasting for the first week or two, but your body will adapt and your appetite will naturally decrease during your feeding times. This is because when you get used to using up all of the food you consumed in your previous eating window (this takes about twelve hours, by the way), the transition from using glucose to ketones as fuel is triggered. Ketones are a natural appetite suppressant.

Perhaps you've heard that the calories you eat actually never matter when you start intermittent fasting. Well, they do, but not in the typical calorie-counting way you're used to. It's more about the *quality* of the calories you take in than the *quantity*.

If you eat primarily healthful, nutrient-dense whole foods, a wide variety of vegetables and whole grains, nuts, legumes, healthy fats, eggs and other proteins (animal or plant-based), you will likely be satisfied before you eat to the point of weight-gain-inducing overconsumption. If you make all your own food, you also probably don't have to count calories.

However, if you fill your feasting window with highly processed foodstuffs, take-out, pizza, doughnuts, and so on, Houston, we may have a problem—at least in the beginning. It's in the beginning that you most need small wins to convince you to stay the course. Eating junk food will cause you to have a harder time adjusting to IF while also not giving you the nutrition that you need.

How Long Will It Take to See Results?

The answer is that it depends on what results you're looking for. You will see improvements to your fasting blood glucose the very first fast you do. You will likely see changes in your waist circumference within a week and feel more energy and less pain (if you are suffering from any) within two weeks. Most people, though not everyone, will see numbers on the scale move within the first week.

This is why I recommend taking measurements and photos on day one and at regular (weekly or bi-weekly) intervals as you go along and stick with it for at least a month. IF is a lifestyle that has been proven to be amazing for weight loss, but there are so many additional non-scale health victories that should not be discounted. Long-term insulin resistance and/or other hormonal issues can make your initial efforts feel very slow to realize results. Don't give up.

Why Am I Losing Inches When the Scale Isn't Moving?

This ties into taking photos and measurements regularly. If you are losing inches but not pounds, there is a good chance that one of two things is going on:

- **Your body is going through recomposition. You are losing fat, which takes up a lot of volume, and gaining muscle tissue, which is denser than fat. This is great! Muscle burns more calories than fat, and you are increasing your resting metabolic rate while looking leaner and fitter!**

- **You have been suffering from chronic inflammation without realizing it, and that is going away with your dietary changes. Also great! Inflammation is both the precursor to and result of illness. Reduced inflammation = improved health.**

If you are sticking to the plan for a month, eating nutritiously, and still not seeing movement in measurements *or* the scale, it's probably a good time to check in with your doctor to see whether other hormonal or autoimmune issues are at play.

Is Fasting Different for Women?

The short answer is yes. The difference is not as extreme as many articles based on studies of male and female rats would have you think because mice and rats are not the same as humans. One day of fasting for a rat is more like a week of fasting for a human.

Women have more responsive hormonal systems than men do when it comes to food restriction. Leptin and ghrelin, the satiety and hunger hormones, are much more sensitive in women, so women may feel hungrier than men as they start fasting. Because women of childbearing years have a hormone-based fertility (menstrual) cycle, prolonged food restriction can affect that as well.

This does not mean that women cannot or should not practice intermittent fasting, even in daily form. What it does mean is that during the feasting window, in particular the week before your period, include nutrient-dense carbohydrates such as beans, rice, lentils, squash, potatoes, sweet potatoes, and whole grains. This supports progesterone production and will help keep your cycle (and your mood!) on track while providing the most benefits in conjunction with intermittent fasting.

Slight changes in your cycle are normal when you give your diet an overhaul in any way, shape, or form. If the changes are drastic—you stop getting your period, or you feel chilled all the time, even when you're not fasting—you may want to rethink IF or at least consume additional calories during your eating windows, particularly from starchy carbohydrates. Extended fasts can still be okay, but not during the week before your period (luteal phase).

For women who no longer get their period, it is also a good idea to consume the carbohydrate sources mentioned previously with at least weekly frequency to maintain progesterone levels and keep anxiety down, even if you are otherwise following a low-carbohydrate or ketogenic diet.

Intermittent fasting has been shown to be a very successful strategy for many women to increase their health. We do, however, need to be mindful of our feasting, making sure we consume enough calories *all* the time and enough carbohydrates, particularly in that luteal phase of the menstrual cycle.

What Are "Clean" and "Dirty" Fasting?

"Clean" fasting entails not consuming anything that may cause an insulinogenic (insulin-generating) or anti-autophagic reaction that will hinder the fast. This means drinking only water, unflavored sparkling water, unflavored mineral water, plain black coffee, unsweetened green or black tea, and salt or electrolytes when you are not in your feasting window.

"Dirty" fasting entails consuming zero to very few (50) calories during your fasting period, but what you consume may spike insulin, hinder fat-burning, and stop autophagy. Because it sometimes helps with compliance to IF, it is not completely frowned upon, but it is a slippery slope. A dirty fast may include diet sodas, flavored seltzers, flavored coffees, fruit-based teas, artificially sweetened gum or mints, small amounts of cream or pure fats such as butter or MCT oil, bone broth, and food of any kind.

Dirty fasting, particularly with the consumption of fat and therefore called a "fat fast," may help you last a little longer in your fasting window with little to no insulin spike. In this case, "dirty" is not a dirty word, *especially* because you are working your way into an intermittent fasting lifestyle.

There is also a list of potentially acceptable foods to consume during your fasting window that may even increase autophagy, such as 1 to 2 teaspoons of apple cider vinegar, cinnamon, ginger, or turmeric teas, and water with a slice of lemon or lime. Is it 100 percent "clean"? Not by

definition, but these items are also unlikely to hinder the fasting benefits and certain ones may even increase them.

Are Artificial Sweeteners Okay?

There is not one fasting guru/authority who approves of artificial sweeteners in any way, shape, or form during the fast. Anecdotally, many people continue to have weight-loss success while still enjoying them, but they cause an insulin response, thereby hindering fat loss. Studies show that consumption of artificial sweeteners can have a negative metabolic effect in both humans and rats.

Consuming them during your eating window is like consuming anything else—up to you. If you find yourself hitting a stall, it may be worth cutting out artificial sweeteners and seeing what happens.

What Will Break a Fast?

Technically, *any* calories will break a fast. There are even people who will argue that coffee and tea break a fast and only plain water is a true non-fast breaker. Plain, unsweetened coffee (regular or decaf) and tea are still advocated by just about every fast-promoting doctor and guru because they not only make compliance easier, they also are mild appetite suppressants and energy boosters.

What About Exercise?

Exercise is great and health-promoting! It tones your cardiovascular system and can give you a great physique. Resistance training (weight-bearing exercises) will help you increase muscle mass at a faster pace, thereby helping you increase your basal metabolic rate and burn more calories in a day. Gentle to moderate exercise also stimulates the lymphatic system, through which triglycerides (broken down fat) are moved to provide the body with energy when glucose is in short supply, such as when you're fasting.

That said, introducing a new or intense exercise regime while you are adapting to intermittent fasting will likely make you hungrier and thus work against you. My recommendation is to get used to fasting before increasing the level of exercise that your body normally gets.

Experienced fasters are able to accomplish all sorts of exercise-related feats; I read about a woman in one of the online fasting groups I belong to who had run 20 miles (32 km) fasted without "hitting the wall"! Take the time to get used to your new fasting lifestyle and *then* incorporate more physical activity.

Is My Hair Going to Fall Out from Fasting?

Any significant dietary change may result in hair loss around the three- to six-month mark, but it doesn't necessarily happen to everyone. If you start noticing significant hair loss outside of this time, it is more likely that you are not getting enough calories and nutrients. When you are in your feasting windows, do not be excessively restrictive of your calories. Make sure you are eating at least to your basal metabolic rate (BMR).

Troubleshooting: When Should I Stop Fasting?

If you experience any of the following symptoms, stop fasting and seek professional medical advice, especially if you have a pre-existing health condition:

- **Dizziness despite electrolyte supplementation and hydration**
- **Consistent nausea**
- **Vomiting**
- **Disorientation**
- **Prolonged fatigue or exhaustion**

Fasting is an amazing tool for most people to improve health, but if you seem to be going in the other direction, it might not be for *you*. That is okay, too. Take care of your health—IF is a method you can always try at another time of your life.

CHAPTER FOUR

Next Level Hacks

We've discussed the physical aspect of intermittent fasting up to this point, but more than half the journey is actually about mindset. Repeating the physical habits will *eventually* make sticking to your IF plan automatic, but how do you stay focused in the beginning, when it's so easy to get distracted and your hormones aren't cooperating yet? There are several tools available to you, all of which count as forms of self-care and most of which come at low-to-no cost.

Food Journaling/Tracking

Keeping a record of what you eat is one of the most proven ways to stay on track, whether you do it in a notebook, via an app, or by taking photos with your phone. This is particularly helpful in the beginning for anyone getting used to the concept of IF who overeats when their feeding window opens. If you are doing alternate daily fasting in particular, it can be very easy to surpass 500 to 600 calories when that eating window comes around!

Sometimes people drastically *undereat* in an effort to speed weight loss, and that can backfire in a big way, too, causing the adaptive thermogenesis we mentioned in the beginning. This lowers the number of calories your body burns at rest and makes it easier to gain weight even though you are eating fewer calories overall. IF is indeed a balance.

Journaling or tracking is a great way to hold yourself accountable, even if the only thing you do is take a quick pic of your plate. Once you're in the swing of things, I guarantee that you will be able to recognize your hunger and satiety signals and eat without tracking or counting calories. If you see the numbers on the scale or measuring tape stop moving, you can always track again.

Meal Planning

We have a chapter of this book devoted to the topic of meal planning (see page 54), but here's the nutshell version why it is so helpful, especially in the beginning: Meal planning is another accountability tool that you can employ before your feast, even if it's just deciding which foods you're going to eat when your window opens and not necessarily preparing them yet.

Hungry minds do not always make the wisest choices! Despite being a chef who has been preparing healthy, nourishing, well-balanced meals for my clients for ages, a desire to satisfy immediate hunger led to a lot of tortillas slathered in mayonnaise over the years and a waistline and booty that would not stop expanding.

Making meal planning a priority changed all of that for me. When I know what I'm planning to eat, and I plan something delicious, it's easy to hold out for it. I even plan when I go to restaurants by checking menus online and it helps get me excited for the meal before it even happens!

You can even write down your meals in your journal before they happen, which is an effective way to stick to your plan because it stimulates the reticular activating system (RAS). The RAS is in the same area of your brain that triggers the fight-or-flight response and is the master player in cognition and decision making. When you write items down before they happen, your subconscious mind is programmed to make the choices that match your written intentions. In fact, you are 40 percent more likely to successfully finish these tasks! How cool is *that*?

Fasting Apps

Much like food-tracking applications, there are multiple free fast-tracking applications, as well, that let you choose the kind of fast you want to do or design your own program. You can set alerts for when your fast ends, connect with other intermittent fasters, and share your progress on social media should you so desire. These apps are a super accountability tool and help keep your eyes off the clock.

Meditation/Mindfulness Practices

Hold on before you skip this section for being too "woo" for you—meditation and mindfulness practices are scientifically proven to help reduce levels of the stress hormone cortisol, also referred to as "the belly fat hormone." Cortisol can stop weight loss in its tracks no matter *what* you're doing right.

Excess cortisol stimulates glucose production. The presence of glucose triggers insulin production. Studies show that increases in cortisol have a corresponding and significant increase in insulin production, more so in women than in men.

Any type of meditation will lower cortisol levels and reduce stress-related anxiety. You do not have to go to a center or do it with a group, though I find that can be an enjoyable experience. You can simply set a timer and sit in stillness with your eyes closed, repeat a mantra, listen to a guided meditation on one of the many free meditation apps out there, count your breaths, try Loving-Kindness Meditation, practice a walking meditation, and so on. There are countless ways to meditate.

There are also countless mindfulness practices available to try, such as breath work and yoga. Studies show that deep diaphragmatic breathing can reduce stress and cortisol levels by stimulating the vagus nerve in the brain, which triggers the parasympathetic response by causing the release of a neurotransmitter called acetylcholine. Acetylcholine sends messages directly to your internal organs to create calm-you-down proteins and enzymes that help release anti-stress hormones such as the feel-good hormone, oxytocin. Yoga, in which breathing also plays an integral role, does the same thing.

Apart from helping regulate your hormones, meditation and mindfulness practices will also help you check in with your body and feelings, possibly helping you decipher true hunger from emotional hunger as you are dealing with cravings and hangriness in the beginning of your journey.

Exercise

In the FAQs (see page 28), I stressed the importance of not undertaking a drastic new exercise regime while adapting to IF, and I stand by that statement. That said, making even a little time for gentle exercise, such as a 10- to 20-minute walk per day, does have stress-lowering and lymphatic-stimulation effects. It also functions as a way to distract yourself and stay busy when you might otherwise feel like eating.

Join IF Support Groups

Whether through Facebook, Reddit, MeetUp, Instagram, one of the fasting apps, or in your local community, there are other people on this journey who are awesome at providing you with inspiration and support when you need a little push to keep going. Join one! Join five! Join however many you feel like. You will likely find other people asking questions that you have, too, and get the opportunity to watch others' health transformations as you are going through your own. You might even make a friend or two.

Get Enough Sleep

Poor sleep is linked to obesity. Research shows that poor sleep results in decreased glucose tolerance, decreased insulin sensitivity, and decreased levels of leptin. It also shows increased evening concentrations of cortisol, increased levels of ghrelin, and increased hunger and appetite. Lack of sleep seems to cause people to make poorer food choices as the reward centers of the brain are activated to a higher level by food when you are sleep deprived.

There are actually so many studies connecting poor sleep with negative health consequences that I could write an entire chapter on this topic, but let's get to the important information: the magic number for healthful sleep seems to be seven to nine hours per night. Start practicing good sleep hygiene:

- **Cut caffeine consumption by the late afternoon.**

- **If it's possible, make sure your feasting window closes at least three hours before bedtime.**

- **Discontinue screen usage one hour before bedtime.**

- **Sleep in a dark room.**

- **Keep your phone outside the bedroom and invest in an inexpensive, small, battery-operated alarm clock to use instead.**

- **Stick to regular wake and sleep times, even on the weekends.**

- **Go to the bathroom before you go to bed.**

- **If it's within your budget, consider upgrading your mattress, or even just pillows that have seen better days.**

This may sound like a challenge with all that is going on in your life, but if you want to gain as many health benefits as possible (as well as the easiest fasting hours ever), it's worth making getting enough sleep a priority.

CHAPTER FIVE

Goal Setting! Knowing Your Numbers and Designing Your Fasting Plan

Are you ready to get this fasting party started? It's time to choose your plan of attack. Writing down your goals and plans makes you *much* more likely to achieve them.

Fill out the following worksheet and refer to it often in your journey to remind yourself why you started and how far you've come.

Intermittent Fasting Worksheet

Name:

Date:

What Are Your Reasons for Starting Intermittent Fasting?

Take a few minutes to think about how you want IF to work for you. Visualize yourself having succeeded already, in the exact shape, size, and level of health that you desire. How will achieving your goal make you feel?

Using the questions that follow as guides, write down five *specific ways* you will know when you have reached your goal. For instance, instead of "I want to look better," write "I will fit into size X jeans again!" Turn "I want to feel better" into "I can walk farther without pain," "I can run up and down the stairs without getting winded," or "I have enough energy to last me the entire day!"

1. What does success look like?
2. What does success *feel* like?
3. What am I trying to "fix"?
4. What will be the first sign that IF is working for me?
5. How will reaching this goal change my life?

What Intermittent Fasting Method Are You Planning to Use?

You've got to commit and stick with the program for at *least* a month. You can do this! If you're brand-new to intermittent fasting, it may be easier to start with a longer feasting window and start extending your fasting hours once you are used to it.

I plan to start with the _____ method on (enter start date) _____ and commit to (at least four) _____ weeks before switching things up!

TRE: My feasting window will be from _____ a.m./p.m. to _____ a.m./p.m. during the week and from _____ a.m./p.m. to _____ a.m./p.m. on the weekend.

ADF: I intend to fast on (enter days) _____ every week and eat normally on (enter days) _____ .

Starting Measurements

We'll start with the most popular gauge—weight—because weight loss is why many people begin IF. Please be aware in your journey that weight loss is not linear. It may take some time for the scale to match up with the way you are looking and feeling!

Height: _____   Starting weight: _____   Goal weight: _____

Use a soft tape measure for sewing or crafts to take your measurements. These numbers will be your most accurate gauge of progress as they reflect size and composition changes even if the scale seems to be staying the same. I recommend taking measurements at least every other week.

1. Waist (at the belly button for consistency):
2. Hips (widest part of your hips):
3. Arm (left or right, midway between elbow and armpit):
4. Thigh (left or right, midway between groin and knee):
5. Neck (midway between chin and collarbone):
6. Chest (at the nipple for consistency):

Basal Metabolic Rate (BMR) and Total Daily Energy Expenditure (TDEE) Calculation

Basal metabolic rate (BMR) is the minimum number of calories that you should consume during your feasting window. Total daily energy expenditure (TDEE) is the upper limit around which you should stay, particularly if you are practicing time-restricted eating (TRE). There is a little more leeway with alternate daily fasting because you will be restricting your calories every other day, but remember that you will still need an overall weekly caloric deficit to lose weight.

As weight changes, you will occasionally need to recalculate the following numbers! I recommend recalculating every 10 pounds (4.5 kg).

Use the following formula to calculate your BMR:

- **Weight in kilograms = weight in pounds × 2.2**
- **Height in centimeters = height in inches × 0.393**
- **Men: BMR = 66 + (13.7 × weight in kilograms) + (5 × height in centimeters) – (6.8 × age in years)**
- **Women: BMR = 655 + (9.6 × weight in kilograms) + (1.8 × height in centimeters) – (4.7 × age in years)**

MY BMR: _____

To calculate your TDEE: Use the Harris-Benedict equation to factor in your activity level, such as your job, daily routine, and of course, training.

- **Little or no exercise = BMR × 1.2**
- **Lightly active (light exercise/work 1 to 3 days per week) = BMR × 1.375**
- **Moderately active (moderate exercise/work 3 to 5 days per week) = BMR × 1.55**
- **Very active (hard exercise/work 6-7 days a week) = BMR × 1.725**
- **Extra active (very hard exercise/work 6-7 days a week) = BMR × 1.9**

MY TDEE: _____

Body Fat Percentage (%) Calculation

Fat loss is one of the primary goals of intermittent fasting and one of the best ways to track progress.

The most accurate ways of calculating body fat are through water displacement and DEXA scans, but these may be harder to get done depending on where you are located and what resources are available to you. Using your measurements and a calculator, determine your body fat percentage with the U.S. Navy's body fat estimation method. If the equation seems too complex, you can easily find a calculator online where you can plug in your measurements and gender.

For men, use the following formula:
% body fat = 86.010 + log10 (abdomen − neck = [inches]) − 70.041 × log10 (height) + 36.76

For women, use the following formula:
% body fat = 163.205 × log10 (waist + hip − neck = [inches]) − 97.684 × log10 (height) − 78.387

Don't Forget About Non-Scale Victories

As you proceed in your IF journey, there's more to watch for than just falling numbers regarding what we've just calculated. Keep your eyes peeled for any of the following signs of success, which other fasters have experienced, to stay motivated, and know this isn't even a complete list!

- Softer, clearer skin
- Skin tags disappearing
- A healthy glow
- Fewer wrinkles
- Skin tightening
- Reduced stretch marks
- Hair growth/regrowth
- Shiny hair
- Reduced edema
- Better sleep
- Lower HbA1C (The hemoglobin A1C test measures your blood sugar over the previous 2 to 3 months and is often used as a measurement tool for diabetes and diabetes risk.)
- Lower fasting glucose, cholesterol and triglycerides
- Improved blood pressure
- Reduction in chronic pain and symptoms of arthritis
- Increased menstrual regularity and fertility
- Reduced depression and/or anxiety

- Clearer thinking, diminished brain fog
- Reversed fatty liver disease
- Change in scar tissue texture and visibility
- Minimized allergy symptoms
- Reduced irritable bowel syndrome symptoms
- Diminished acid reflux and/or GERD symptoms
- Increased libido
- Sharper senses (eyesight, smell, taste, and so on)
- Decreased hunger
- Increased compliments from friends, family, and strangers!*

* Although this one is one of my personal favorites, bear in mind that the people who see you the most often may not as readily see the gradual changes. That's normal! Seriously, the guy working at the corner store who I see once in a blue moon was giving me high fives way before my closest friends even noticed my IF success!

2

Feasting

"The proof of the pudding is in the eating."

—PROVERB

The fun part is here at last! It's important for you to combine the two components, delicious *and* nutritious, to get the most satisfaction out of every meal. Nourishing your soul with pleasure while you fuel your body with healthy foods will maximize your chances for staying the course and getting the results you want. We're going to talk about the different kinds of deliciousness you'll get to enjoy during the feasting part of this journey. The possibilities are endless, the world is your oyster, so let's get going!

CHAPTER SIX

What We Eat
Still Matters

Chances are, you have been investigating intermittent fasting already and seen claims that you can eat anything you want using IF and still lose weight. That may indeed be true—for *some* people. The fact is, everybody is different, and no two IF journeys will be alike. One person may be fasting for weight loss while another is fasting for stem cell production. This woman may have food allergies or autoimmune conditions to contend with while this man has never found a food that didn't love his body back.

This part of the book teaches you how to efficiently obtain the most nutrition in the reduced amount of time that you have. You are embarking on a fantastic, easy-to-assimilate lifestyle that shortens the time you have to consume all the vitamins and minerals you need. To make up for that, choose colorful, natural, whole food ingredients and/or prepared foods at least 80 percent* of the time.

Choosing these kinds of foods will generally allow you to eat *more*, i.e., a greater quantity, while also feeling more satisfied. The key lies in nutrient density.

*Why 80 percent of the time and not 100 percent? Because we're all human and there's not one perfect one among us. The goal is progress, not perfection, and if you're going to get tied up in guilt or shame for not fasting or feasting perfectly, you're likely not going to stick with it. Plus, sometimes you just want a margarita, right?!

Nutrient Density

Nutrient density refers to foods with a higher quantity of beneficial vitamins, minerals, and amino acids per calorie compared to most other foods. It is often contrasted with energy density, or calorie density, though some foods can be both calorie dense and nutrient dense simultaneously. Understanding how this works requires a basic knowledge of macronutrients and micronutrients.

Macronutrients

There are three categories of macronutrients, often shortened to "macros," when we talk about food. They consist of carbohydrates, protein, and fat. They are the primary suppliers of nutrients in your overall diet.

Carbohydrates

Carbohydrates, or carbs, tend to be the primary source of fuel for the mental and physical processes of the human body. They come in two forms:

- Simple Carbohydrates: These are absorbed quickly into the bloodstream, raising blood glucose and creating an insulin response in a short amount of time. If you've ever experienced a sugar high and its subsequent crash, simple carbohydrates are usually to blame. They include sugar itself, white flour, candy, soda, and so on, and are frequently referred to as empty calories because they provide no actual health benefit to the body.

- Complex Carbohydrates: Consumption of these carbs provides health benefits because they contain fiber and nutrients. Absorption is slower and the rise in blood glucose is lower, as is the corresponding rise in insulin. This category includes fruit, vegetables, legumes, and whole grains.

Macronutrient Quick Guide		
Macronutrient	Calories Per Gram	Function
Carbohydrate	4	Primary source of glucose-based energy as well as fiber to aid digestion.
Protein	4	Composed of amino acids. Provides the building blocks for new proteins, muscle repair, and hormone and enzyme production. Also an energy source.
Fat	9	Supplies fatty acids the body needs but cannot make, such as omega-3s. Assists absorption of fat-soluble vitamins A, D, E, K, and carotenoids. Aids digestion and makes food more palatable.

Protein

Protein has many roles, making up our connective tissue, hair, and muscle and also functioning as immune antibodies, hormones, and enzymes. It is stored primarily in our muscles and not used as a source of energy except in extreme cases. Protein is composed of twenty amino acids, which are broken down into three categories:

- Essential: We can't survive without these amino acids, but our bodies can't produce them, so we *must* obtain them from food sources.

- Semi-essential: The body can produce these but not in sufficient quantities in certain circumstances (such as during childhood or illness), so we must supplement them with food sources.

- Nonessential: The body makes enough of these amino acids without supplementation. Nonessential, however, does not mean not important.

Fat

Thank goodness the tide has changed regarding fat consumption, because fat is incredibly important to our well-being in so many ways! We need fat to absorb fat-soluble vitamins A, D, E, and K. Fat insulates and protects our organs, helps to regulate hormone production, and it makes food taste good and feel more filling, delivering the satiety that we seek.

Fatty acids can be delivered in three primary forms:

- Saturated fats are solid fats found in red meat, coconut oil, lard, butter, and other dairy products such as cream cheese and full-fat cheeses. They've been regarded as unhealthy for decades because they raise levels of low-density lipoproteins (LDL), or "bad," cholesterol in the blood, increasing the risk of heart disease. However, recent studies show that there are two LDL subtypes: (1) small, dense LDL that can penetrate the arterial wall easily, driving heart disease and (2) large, fluffy LDL, which can't breach the arterial wall. Saturated fats have been shown to increase the size of LDL, rendering them benign. They've also been shown to increase healthy, high-density lipoproteins (HDL). There's no need to fear saturated fat.

- Unsaturated fats protect the brain and aid cardio-vascular health, as well as decrease inflammation and help repair injuries. They include *monounsaturated fatty acids*, which are considered healthy fats that have been shown to preserve cardiac health. They are found in sources such as olive oil, avocados, sesame oil, and nuts. *Polyunsaturated fatty acids* are also in the healthy fat category and are important in building nerve coverings and cell membranes. We need them for blood clotting, muscle movement, and preventing inflammation. They come in two types: omega-3 fatty acids and omega-6 fatty acids.

- Trans fats include partially hydrogenated, ultra-refined fat sources such as margarine and most shortenings. Trans fats are unhealthy and should be avoided. They have been shown to increase the small, dense, and harmful LDL, but unlike saturated fats, they do not result in a corresponding increase in HDL. Trans fats have been linked to increases in heart disease.

Micronutrients

Micronutrients are nutrients we need in minute amounts, but we require more than thirty different ones for our bodies to function normally. We need them for immunity, brainpower (clear thinking), skin health, metabolic function, energy levels, and also stress mitigation. Deficiencies can lead to serious and chronic diseases, potentially taking years from our lives.

Micronutrients consist of vitamins and minerals. Our bodies cannot produce them on their own, so we *must* get all of our micronutrients from food. This is more of a challenge in today's world as intensive commercial farming practices have stripped the soil of increasing amounts of nutrients, meaning that fruits and vegetables do not have the same nutrient profiles as they did even fifty years ago. This is also why eating foods that are as nutrient dense as possible is integral to a healthy body.

Micronutrient Quick Guide

Micronutrient	Function	Where Found	Signs Of Deficiency
Vitamin A	Promotes strong bones and teeth, good eyesight and healthy skin	Liver, fish oil, tomatoes, dark leafy greens, oranges	Skin problems, itchiness, poor night vision
Vitamin B$_1$ (thiamine)	Supports carbohydrate metabolism	Whole grains, nuts, organ meats, eggs	Muscle fatigue, reduced reflexes, blurry vision, irritability, tingling in arms and legs, nausea
Vitamin B$_3$ (Niacin)	Maintains nervous system; metabolizes carbohydrates and fat; produces sex hormones	Organ meats, poultry, dry beans and legumes, nuts	Sun rash, low sex drive, apathy, depression, headache, fatigue, disorientation
Vitamin B$_{12}$	Produces new blood cells in bone marrow; supports nervous system	Organ meats, red meat, poultry, dairy, eggs	Fatigue, anemia, palpitations, breathlessness
Vitamin B$_9$ (folate)	Produces red blood cells; supports cell division, DNA production, and healthy pregnancy	Dark leafy greens, egg yolks, whole grains, nuts	Headaches, irritability, difficulty concentrating, shortness of breath
Vitamin B$_2$ (riboflavin)	Supports endocrine system; aids digestive process; repairs injured tissue	Eggs, brown rice, organ meats, dark leafy greens, Brewer's yeast	Mouth sores, cracks at corners of mouth, inflamed tongue
Vitamin C	Antioxidant; boosts immunity; supports healthy skin and bones	Citrus fruits, red vegetables, kiwi, green vegetables	Rough and/or dry skin, fatigue, sore and/or bleeding gums, painful, swollen joints, delayed wound healing, bruising, spoon-shaped fingernails
Vitamin D	Regulates calcium for bone health	Sunlight, fortified dairy, eggs, organ meats	Osteoporosis, liver and kidney issues, depression, hair loss, bone and back pain, weak immune system
Vitamin E	Bolsters red blood cells; promotes wound healing; protects against heart disease, cataracts, macular degeneration	Liver, eggs, nuts, seeds, cold-pressed vegetable oils, sweet potatoes, asparagus, dark leafy greens, avocado	Brittle hair, dry skin, bruising, hot flashes, eczema, psoriasis, cataracts, delayed wound healing, muscle weakness, anemia, PMS
Calcium	Builds bones and teeth; promotes muscle movement and cell function	Dairy, molasses, Brazil nuts, broccoli, cabbage, dark leafy greens, hazelnuts, oysters, sardines, canned salmon	Osteoporosis, osteoarthritis, muscle cramps, anxiety, increased colon cancer risk

Micronutrient Quick Guide

Micronutrient	Function	Where Found	Signs Of Deficiency
Magnesium	Builds bones and teeth; aids nervous system, heart rhythm, immune system; regulates calcium, copper, zinc, potassium, vitamin D	Green vegetables, dry beans, nuts, seeds, whole grains, avocado	Increased appetite, nausea, fatigue cramps, numbness, tingling, heart rhythm issues
Iron	Transports oxygen to the red blood cells and muscles	Leafy greens, nuts, seaweed, whole grains, liver, meat, sardines	Anemia, chronic fatigue, paleness, shortness of breath
Zinc	Lowers blood sugar; supports immune system, prostate gland, and sperm production	Oysters, red meat, poultry, nuts, seafood, whole grains, dairy	Hair loss, diarrhea, impotence, slowed wound healing, mental lethargy
Chromium	Assists insulin function; increases fertility; supports carbohydrate and fat metabolism	Seafood, meat, whole grains, broccoli, prunes, nuts, potatoes	Metabolic syndrome, insulin resistance, decreased fertility
Selenium	Antioxidant; works with vitamin E; supports prostaglandins production, thyroid function; increases fertility; helps cognitive function	Brazil nuts, sunflower seeds, liver, butter, shellfish, cold water fish, whole grains	Heart and pancreas problems, sore muscles, weakened immune system, weakened red blood cells
CoQ$_{10}$	Antioxidant; supports healthy cholesterol, heart, liver, and kidneys	Fatty fish, organ meats, whole grains	Congestive heart failure, high blood pressure, gingivitis, heart arrhythmia
Carnitine	Helps metabolize ketones; supports energy, heart function	Red meat, dairy, fish, poultry, tempeh, avocados, asparagus, peanuts, peanut butter	High cholesterol, poor liver function, muscle weakness, impaired glucose control, reduced energy
N-acetyl-L-cysteine and glutathione	Supports eye, lung, and immune system health; liver detoxification; anti-inflammatory; decreases muscle fatigue	Meats, ricotta cheese, yogurt, wheat germ, oats	Increases cancer risk, potential of cataracts and macular degeneration, reduces immune response
Alpha lipoic acid	Supports insulin sensitivity, effectiveness of vitamins C and E; increases energy	Spinach, broccoli, beef, seeds	Diabetic neuropathy, reduced muscle mass, increases Alzheimer's risk
Copper	Aids in bone formation; active in healing processes; stimulates iron absorption; assists fatty acid metabolism	Oysters, seeds, dark leafy greens, organ meats, dry beans, nuts, shellfish, whole grains, chocolate, soybeans, oats, blackstrap molasses	Osteoporosis, anemia, hair loss, impaired lung functions, decreased immunity

Electrolytes

Electrolytes are a particular kind of micronutrient that are *incredibly* important to our health and well-being. They are specific minerals that carry an electric charge when mixed with water (our bodies are 75 percent water, by the way), and our bodies need them to function. Electrolytes keep our cells, tissues, and fluids communicating within our bodies. They are essential for heart health, brain functioning, and muscle contraction.

Maintaining electrolyte levels keeps us hydrated, feeling good, thinking clearly, and able to make it through the day. As your body adapts to intermittent fasting, it changes the way it handles water and electrolytes, often flushing out more through the kidneys than usual. Our bodies produce less insulin and dip into glycogen reserves in the liver. Water and stored electrolytes are released through urine, sweat, and the breath. This means that we must try to ensure that we are getting enough from food sources and supplementation to make up for those mineral losses.

The primary electrolytes we need to pay attention to are sodium, potassium, magnesium, calcium, and chloride.

Sodium. Sodium regulates the total amount of water in the body and is found in blood, lymph, and plasma fluid. It maintains the balance *outside* the cell, though it plays an important role in transmitting signals among the brain, nervous system, and muscles. We need 4,000–7,000 mg per day while fasting and good sources include: table salt, Himalayan salt, sea salt, pickles, tomato juices, broths, and soups.

Potassium. Potassium is integral for fluid balance *within* the cells and is required for normal cell function. Potassium regulates the heartbeat and blood pressure and is needed for all muscle function. We need 2,000–4,700 mg per day while fasting and whole food sources are ideal to prevent getting *too* much. Sources include potatoes, bananas, avocados, coconut water, Brussels sprouts, spinach, mushrooms, zucchini, fatty fish, beef, oysters, and pork. You can stay on the lower end of the scale if you are not exercising intensely.

Magnesium. Magnesium is also a key component in hormone regulation, muscle pain alleviation, and managing, if not preventing, sugar cravings. We need it for nerve and muscle function, muscle development, blood sugar regulation and blood pressure maintenance. Per day, women need 320 mg and men need 420 mg while fasting. Good sources include brazil nuts, dark leafy greens, cacao and dark chocolate, pumpkin seeds, almonds and other nuts, mackerel, and pollock. Because it is a little more challenging to get all the magnesium we need from food sources, this electrolyte is worth supplementing.

Calcium. Most of our calcium is stored in our bones, which the body taps into when cellular and/or muscular supplies run low. Calcium is necessary for blood clotting, normal heart rhythm, muscle contraction, and formation of bones and teeth. We need 1,000 mg per day while fasting, and this can be achieved by consuming dark leafy greens, sardines, dairy products, broccoli, almonds, and chia seeds.

Quick Electrolyte Guide		
Electrolyte	**Daily requirement**	**Best sources**
Sodium	4,000–7,000 mg	2 teaspoons salt per day; Himalayan or sea salt to get the highest amount of trace minerals
Potassium	2,000–4,700 mg	Avocados, coconut water, bananas, No-Salt or Lite salt
Magnesium	320–420 mg	Dark leafy greens, spinach, almonds, fish, chocolate
Calcium	1,000 mg	Dairy, chia seeds, dark leafy greens, sesame seeds

Eating the Rainbow

I have long advised my clients to eat "a rainbow" every day, meaning consuming plant foods of various colors. The colors of various plant foods are indicators of the kinds of beneficial micronutrients and antioxidants they contain.

Red and pink fruits and vegetables such as grapefruit, strawberries, red peppers, watermelon, beets, and tomatoes contain a rock star antioxidant called lycopene from the carotenoid family as well as vitamins A and C. Lycopene may have protective properties against sunburn, helps reduce the risk of or even slows the growth of certain cancers, and promotes a healthy heart. Tomatoes are extra nutritious and packed with B vitamins.

Orange and yellow fruits and veggies contain different kinds of carotenoids than lycopene. Beta carotene, another powerful antioxidant, is a precursor of vitamin A (retinol), meaning that it is converted in the body only at levels the body requires. Vitamin A helps maintain healthy skin, mucous membranes, and vision. Lutein, another carotenoid orange and yellow fruits and vegetables possess, is another antioxidant that has been shown to prevent cataracts and age-related macular degeneration, which can lead to blindness.

Green vegetables such as leafy greens and Brussels sprouts contain a range of phytochemicals including carotenoids, indoles, and saponins, all of which have anticancer properties. They also tend to be loaded with folate and vitamins A, C, and K, which is enormously important to blood and bone health.

Purple and blue fruits and veggies (and even grains such as black rice) get their vivid hues from a plant pigment called anthocyanin. Anthocyanins have antioxidant properties that have been shown to protect cells from damage and may even help reduce the risk of cancer, stroke, and heart disease. Black rice anthocyanins have been shown in certain studies to induce apoptosis (programmed cell death) and inhibit cancer cell growth.

White and brown fruits and vegetables such as potatoes, cauliflower, turnips, onions, parsnips, mushrooms, garlic, and kohlrabi contain a range of health-promoting phytochemicals. Garlic and onions (both in the allium family) contain a phytochemical called allicin known for its antiviral and antibacterial properties. Both potatoes and bananas are known to be fantastic sources of potassium.

What's In A Plant?	
Polyphenols	Protective compounds in plants that protect us, too! Lower inflammation and help prevent disease.
Antioxidants	Anti-inflammatory compounds that inhibit oxidation, scavenging harmful free radicals in the body.
Flavonoids	Plant-based chemicals, a.k.a. phytonutrients, with some of the greatest antioxidant and anti-inflammatory effects.
Carotenoids	Plant pigments that give fruits and vegetables their red, orange, and yellow colors. Act as anti-inflammatory antioxidants that provide anti-aging benefits.
Tannins	Polyphenols that give many plants and plant products their dark red and brown colors. Think coffee, tea, wine, and chocolate!
Organosulfur compounds	Sulfur-containing compounds that have powerful antioxidant and anti-inflammatory effects and give certain vegetables, such as cauliflower, broccoli, garlic, onions, mustard greens, and horseradish a sharper, stinky odor when cooked.

Color	Contains	Function	Where found
Red and pink	Vitamins A and C, manganese, antioxidants (quercetin, lycopene)	Reduce risk of cancer and heart disease; decrease inflammation; increase immunity; great for eye, skin, and hair health	Tomatoes, berries, cherries, beets, radishes, grapefruit, watermelon, red apples, red potatoes, red peppers
Orange and yellow	Vitamins A, B6, C, potassium, folate, antioxidants (beta-carotene, alpha-carotene, lutein)	Promotes healthy joints and collagen formation; boosts immune system; decreases blood pressure; builds healthier bones working with calcium and magnesium; reduces cancer risk; great for eye, skin, and hair health	Carrots, pumpkin, squash, sweet potatoes, oranges, bananas, apricots, cantaloupe, orange and yellow peppers, peaches, nectarines
Green	Vitamin K, B vitamins, folate, potassium, antioxidants, chlorophyll, carotenoids, lutein	Increase liver function; healthy cell production; lung health; help with blood clotting; lower blood pressure; reduce cancer risk	Broccoli, cabbage, cucumbers, leafy greens, fresh herbs, asparagus, green beans, peas, zucchini, avocado, kiwi, green apples, green grapes, pears, green peppers, okra, romanesco, broccolini
Blue and purple	B vitamins, antioxidants (anthocyanins, resveratrol, flavonoids)	Prevent aging; improve memory; protect cells from damage; reduce cancer and heart disease risks	Eggplant, red onions, purple cabbage, purple potatoes, blueberries, blackberries, plums, purple carrots, purple cauliflower, black grapes
White and brown	Vitamins C and K, folate, potassium, antioxidants (allicin, quercetin, anthoxanthins)	Lower cholesterol and blood pressure; protect cells from damage; increase immune function; reduce cardiovascular and cancer risks; promote eye, skin, and bone health	Cauliflower, garlic, potatoes, parsnips, turnips, rutabaga (swede), mushrooms, onions, leeks, jicama, kohlrabi, horseradish, daikon

Anti-Inflammatory Foods

Intermittent fasting has been shown to reduce chronic inflammation without negatively affecting the body's healthy and necessary inflammatory responses to acute situations. This is why so many practitioners experience reduced pain and alleviation of other symptoms of chronic diseases. You can boost the anti-inflammatory nature of IF by choosing foods that also are known to combat inflammation.

It should come as no surprise, especially given the rest of this chapter, that the top anti-inflammatory foods are some of the most nutrient dense *and* colorful, to boot. They are also among the most delicious, which is why you'll find so many of them included in the recipe section of this book!

Incorporating as many anti-inflammatory foods as you can into your feasting windows will boost your micronutrient consumption, of which even non-fasters are falling short all over the world. More of the following foods will not necessarily *cure* what ails you, but they may help you

- Recover more quickly from exercise-related injuries
- Achieve greater cardiovascular protection than low-fat diets
- Treat chronic skin conditions such as psoriasis
- Reduce depression risks and symptoms

There are many other studies that could be referenced, but that little list should give you an idea of how making the most nutrient-dense food choices can positively influence various aspects of your health. I encourage you to try and include at least one item—and preferably multiple choices—from the foods in the following list in *every* meal you eat. The fewer meals you eat, the more selections you should try to include in your window. Doing this will provide your body with much-needed nutrients and may also offset the pro-inflammatory nature of other foods you might be consuming.

There is one caveat here. Although the foods listed are known and shown to have anti-inflammatory properties, food allergies and intolerances may not make that true for *you*. If you know you are allergic to a food listed below,

don't eat it. If it makes you break out in a rash, turn red, or swell up, or make your joints ache, or gives you a sore belly or stuffy nose, or otherwise makes you feel physically bad, *don't eat it.* These are all pro-inflammatory reactions, though not a complete list by far.

So, what are the top anti-inflammatory foods you can possibly eat?

Berries, Cherries, and Red Grapes — All berries, red grapes, and cherries are super antioxidant rich. Red berries are packed with immune-system-supporting vitamin C, and the darker berries and cherries contain the anthocyanins noted in the section about blue and purple produce (see page 44). Grapes, red wine, and berries also contain resveratrol, a polyphenol that decreases inflammatory free radicals. Cherries contain catechins, another powerful antioxidant we find in more foods on this list and are linked to a whole *heap* of health benefits, such as improved heart health and potentially weight loss.

Fatty Fish — All seafood is a great source of protein and inflammation-reducing omega-3 fatty acids. Salmon, sardines, mackerel, herring, trout, and anchovies are particularly high in EPA and DHA, the long-chain omega-3s that are hailed as being among the most potent anti-inflammatory substances on earth, super heart healthy, and showing great promise in alleviating the pain of rheumatoid arthritis. Wild-caught options provide the highest concentration of omega-3s, but if farmed is your only option, buy it—or take a fish oil supplement. If the fish mentioned are a little on the strong side for you, halibut is a milder tasting option that still has a great concentration, too.

Coffee — I'll bet you didn't see this one coming, but it does come with guidelines. Studies show that consuming up to 5 cups (that's five 8-ounce cups for a total of 40 ounces or 1.1 L) of coffee per day can have multiple health benefits, from decreasing the risk of type 2 diabetes, cardiovascular disease, Alzheimer's, Parkinson's, and certain cancers to increasing memory and athletic performance. Coffee contains polyphenols, plant-based antioxidants that may protect against inflammation and even metabolic syndrome.

Green Tea — Like cherries, all tea (black, white, and green from the *Camellia sinensis* plant) contains catechins, super fabulous antioxidants that reduce inflammation. Green tea has the highest concentration of EGCG, the most potent of the free-radical scavenging catechins, which work in concert with the alkaloids, caffeine, and theobromine, and additional polyphenols to make it an anti-inflammatory superstar. Plus it's fat-burning!

Ginger – Ginger contains a bioactive compound called gingerol (another phenol) that has intensely beneficial medicinal properties. Ginger has been proven to have anticancer, anti-inflammatory, and antioxidant properties, among others. It is also purported to increase autophagy, one of our favorite side-effects of intermittent fasting!

Turmeric – Turmeric is that bright yellow spice you now see in the pharmacy aisle as often as the spice aisle, and with good reason: it contains another super strong anti-inflammatory component called curcumin that has been linked to arthritis relief (by decreasing joint inflammation) and as a potential treatment for cancer.

You can include turmeric in plenty of yummy recipes, but it may be hard to get enough through food alone to reap the benefits. This is a good compound to supplement. When combined with black pepper, which can boost absorption by 2000 percent, it causes a significant decrease in the inflammatory marker C-reactive protein in people with metabolic syndrome.

Leafy Greens – Eat your greens! There's a lot to love about dark leafy greens. Most people think spinach, kale, collards, Swiss chard, arugula, and other lettuces but forget that fresh herbs count here, too! That's right—parsley, cilantro, basil, chervil, and the like are also ultra-nutritious and have anti-inflammatory properties, even if we tend to eat them in smaller amounts. In the course of your day, every little bit counts. The darker the green, the more nutrients, but they all contain vitamins A, C, and K. Spinach contains kaempferol, a pretty special compound that exhibits anticancer properties along with antioxidant, anti-inflammatory, antimicrobial, and antidiabetic ones, as well.

Dark Chocolate and Cocoa – I don't know what's more satisfying—eating chocolate or finding out it's good for you, too! Choose dark chocolate that contains at least 70 percent cocoa to reap the anti-inflammatory benefits of the polyphenols and flavonoids that make it magic. Dark chocolate and cocoa have proven to modulate inflammation in people at risk of cardiovascular disease. They also keep the cells that line your blood vessels, arteries, and lymphatic vessels healthy.

Peppers – Peter Piper must have been one healthy guy. All peppers, whether sweet or hot, have heaps of anti-inflammatory properties. Sweet peppers, in particular the red ones, contain tons of vitamin C, beta carotene, and more anti-inflammatory polyphenols. Milder chile peppers such as poblano and banana peppers reduce inflammation with their high content of sinapic and ferulic acid, also reducing oxidative stress caused by scavenging free radicals. Hot peppers such as jalapeños, serranos, habaneros, Thai bird's eye chiles, and more contain capsaicin, a compound that fights inflammation both when consumed *and* when applied externally. (Note: Wear gloves or wash your hands thoroughly afterward before you touch your eyes or any other sensitive areas.)

Nuts and Seeds – Nuts and seeds, particularly chia, flax, and hemp, are amazing little packages of nutrients and short-chain omega-3s such as alpha-linolenic acid (ALA). The body has to convert ALA to DHA or EPA for it to become active and anti-inflammatory, so it's not as effective as getting the straight stuff from fish sources, but it's still beneficial. Nuts have plenty of other nutritious benefits to make the nosh worth it. Walnuts in particular lead the pack in ALA levels, though other nuts contain them. Walnuts, almonds, and hazelnuts have been shown to be great for brain health and preventative of Alzheimer's, which has recently been called type 3 diabetes.

Chia seeds are rich in vitamins A, B, D, and E and important minerals such as magnesium. They've been shown to help regulate cholesterol, lower blood pressure, and decrease C-reactive protein. Flaxseeds are super high in fiber, which encourages the growth of healthy inflammation-reducing gut bacteria. Hemp hearts (or hemp seeds) are great sources of ALA, protein, vitamins, and minerals.

Extra-Virgin Olive Oil and Coconut Oil – Extra-virgin olive oil is the cornerstone of the famous, anti-inflammatory Mediterranean diet. It contains monounsaturated fatty acids such as inflammation-lowering oleic acid. It is also rich in the antioxidant, cancer-fighting quercetin and the compound oleocanthal, which shares the same anti-inflammatory properties as ibuprofen. Oleocanthal has also been linked to a lower risk of heart disease, degenerative brain disorders, and multiple types of cancer.

Virgin, unrefined coconut oil is a healthy saturated fat that contains high levels of similar inflammation-reducing antioxidants. It has also been shown to have beneficial effects on arthritis. Consuming healthy fats also makes some of the micronutrients we need more bioavailable, so drizzle and sizzle, friends!

Tomatoes — We talked about the antioxidant and anti-inflammatory magic of tomatoes' lycopene and vitamin C in "Eating the Rainbow" (see page 43). Lycopene inhibits both the inflammatory response and obesity resulting from high-fat diets. It's also been shown to increase insulin sensitivity, something many of us are striving for with intermittent fasting. Tomatoes are also rich in potassium, which flushes toxins from the body and helps to regulate blood pressure.

Avocado Avocados, much like olive oil, are excellent sources of monounsaturated fatty acids, which we already know are anti-inflammatory and great for your ticker. They also are great sources of magnesium, potassium, fiber, carotenoids, and tocopherols—in other words, they are nutritional powerhouses.

Broccoli and Its Cruciferous Cousins Cruciferous vegetables in the *brassica* family, among them broccoli, kale, cauliflower, Romanesco, cabbage, bok choy, Brussels sprouts, watercress, collard greens, arugula, radishes, and mustard greens, contain an anti-inflammatory antioxidant called sulforaphane.

Sulforaphane has proven to reduce inflammation, oxidative stress, and harmful advanced glycation end product-induced inflammation (AGE). (AGE form in foods, particularly when cooked at high temperatures. Your body can naturally eliminate small amounts, but larger accumulations over time have been linked to the development of diabetes, kidney issues, heart disease, and premature aging.) Broccoli has the largest amount, but all of the brassicas have it. They also contain cancer-fighting glucosinolates, vitamin K, flavonoids, carotenoids, potassium, magnesium, and tons

of fiber. This is why you will find so many recipes involving one brassica or another in this book!

Dry Beans and Legumes — Research shows that they *are* anti-inflammatory, and they tend to be high in nutrients such as fiber, magnesium, B-complex vitamins, vitamin K, and antioxidant-rich polyphenols. Adding beans such as navy, kidney, pinto, black beans, and garbanzo, plus lentils and split peas to your diet will boost your protein intake. Research also suggests beans may have anti-diabetic, anticarcinogenic, anti-obesity, and heart-protective properties.

Garlic and Onions — Just the smell of garlic and onions cooking puts me in a relaxed, happy place. Yet the nutritional makeup of this family of plants, known as alliums, also makes them highly desirable. They are anti-inflammatory and contain properties that combat depression, hypertension, and potentially cancer. Alliums, which include garlic, onions, shallots, chives, leeks, and green onions, all contain an organosulfur compound called allicin. Allicin has an anti-inflammatory effect and has also been shown to boost the immune system.

Now you know why every recipe in this book contains at least one of the foods listed previously. If your body tolerates these tasty ingredients, it is definitely worthwhile to incorporate at least one of them into every single meal you eat—or at least 80 percent of them!

Feeling Full

One of the biggest issues we all face when embarking on a particular eating plan or diet is feeling full and satisfied when we eat. This is true also for intermittent fasting, though the body soon adjusts and feels fuller faster. How we deal with that less-than-full feeling can be the deal breaker in how long we stay on track.

Your full feeling has more to do with hormone signaling than what you eat. The body produces the satiety hormone leptin, which tells us when we are full (i.e., have consumed enough energy or have enough in storage) and should stop eating. Leptin is produced in fat cells, so you would think that people with more fat would experience less hunger. However, because of factors such as chronic raised insulin and systemic inflammation, cells can become leptin resistant and no longer be able to communicate the feeling of fullness effectively.

Another hormone, mentioned previously several times, is ghrelin. Ghrelin tells us when we *are* hungry and overproducing it in balance with leptin gives us an inaccurate picture of how hungry we really are.

How do we work with that and harness leptin sensitivity once again? By retraining the insulin, ghrelin, and leptin feedback loops. We can do that by sticking to intermittent fasting as well as choosing the right foods, exercising moderately, and getting enough sleep, which is crucial to your hormone signaling.

High Satiety Foods

Extra-filling foods have several common characteristics based on the "Satiety Index" created in 1995 by Susanna Holt, Ph.D., and reported in the *European Journal of Clinical Nutrition*. All of the thirty-eight foods analyzed tended to be:

- **High in protein. Studies show that protein is the most filling macronutrient. It changes the levels of several satiety hormones, including ghrelin.**

- **High in fiber. Fiber provides bulk and helps you feel full for longer. Fiber slows down the emptying of the stomach and increases digestion time.**

- **High in volume. Some foods contain a lot of water or air. They literally fill you up and trigger your stomach-stretch signals that make it uncomfortable to eat more.**

- **Low in energy density. This means that a food is low in calories for its weight. Foods with a low energy density are more filling because they typically contain a lot of water and fiber but are lower in fat.**

Whole, unprocessed foods are generally more filling than processed foods. Nutrient-dense foods, including the anti-inflammatory list we just looked at (see page 45), tend to be more filling than low-nutritive foods.

The Best Foods to Eat to Suppress Appetite for the Longest

Boiled Potatoes — Surprised? I certainly was, but boiled potatoes top the Satiety Index for the most filling food. Cooked, unpeeled potatoes are actually full of nutrients, low in calories, high in volume, and contain moderate amounts of protein and fiber. Bonus—cooking and cooling potatoes creates an even more health-promoting effect because much of the carbohydrate content is converted to resistant starch in the cooling process, a gut-bacteria-feeding prebiotic that causes less of an insulinogenic response.

Fish — Fish came in second on the Satiety Index. In a study comparing satiety after consumption of fish, chicken, and beef, fish was the winner, likely because it includes a lot of protein for relatively low caloric density and plenty of hunger-taming omega-3 fatty acids.

Oatmeal — Oats come in third place on the Satiety Index, primarily for their high fiber content and their high volume due to their ability to soak up water. They actually decrease the insulin response, too.

Soup — Soups provide a greater feeling of satiety than non-liquid meals made from the same exact ingredients. This is true in particular for smooth, pureed soups though the effect is still notable in chunky soups.

Eggs — Eggs are protein rich and nutrient dense while also being relatively low in calories. They raise blood sugar very little, keeping glucose and corresponding insulin levels in check. Studies show that choosing eggs as a breakfast food may lower caloric consumption for the following 36 hours.

Meat – High in protein, meat has a high positive effect on fullness. Choosing leaner cuts also decreases energy density.

Greek Yogurt – Greek yogurt is higher in protein than regular yogurt and higher in volume due to its thick nature. Choosing a higher fat option may also have a more pleasant effect on the palate.

Beans and Legumes – As mentioned previously, beans and legumes are chock-full of fiber, protein, and micronutrients. They also have a high water content, translating to a high volume in relation to calories.

Fruits and Vegetables – High in fiber and volume, low in calories, and packed with micronutrients, it's no wonder that fruits and vegetables make the list. The key is to enjoy the *whole* fruit or vegetable to gain the satiety benefit as the fiber plays a huge role. Apples and oranges have shown higher fullness effects than other fruit.

Popcorn – Popcorn has a lot of fiber, high volume, and very few calories compared to other snack foods. The caveat is that you want to choose air-popped or homemade popcorn to avoid additives and extra calories.

Coconut and MCT Oil – Coconut oil is a bit of an outlier in this list because it does not follow the "rules" of being high fiber, high volume, high protein, or low in calories. That said, something unique to coconut oil is its concentration of medium-chain triglycerides (MCT). MCT have been shown to increase satiety and decrease subsequent food intake, especially when consumed in pure liquid form.

There has been some discussion about the part that fat plays in satiety. Fat makes food more pleasurable to eat, makes certain vitamins and minerals more accessible to the body, and plays a role in delaying gastric emptying. That last part means fat helps keep food in your stomach for longer, making you feel full for longer. Studies show that it is only when foods are high fat in conjunction with high carbohydrate—shelf-stable snack cakes, ribs slathered in sweet barbecue sauces, pastry items—that they can work against you over time. Healthy fats on their own can actually act as appetite suppressants.

Complementary Diet Patterns

The great thing about intermittent fasting is that it does not require changing *how* you eat, only *when* you eat. You don't have to give up any particular foods or food groups. If you have pizza every Friday, you can still have pizza every Friday. If you like to eat something sweet every day, you can still have something sweet every day. If you are vegetarian, gluten-free, lactose-intolerant, allergic to peaches, whatever—nobody is telling you to change your ways! You can still gain health benefits with IF, regardless of what you choose to eat, provided that you are staying in a caloric deficit and sticking to foods you are not intolerant of or allergic to. That said, there are ways of eating that may boost and/or speed up the results you are seeking.

Mediterranean Diet
You have probably heard of the Mediterranean diet as it has been the darling of the cardiovascular care community for a long time. The foundation of the Mediterranean diet is plant-based, loaded with vegetables, fruits, whole grains, and healthy fats from nuts, olives, and olive oil. Weekly consumption of eggs, fish, poultry, and legumes is encouraged, along with more limited intake of red meat and dairy. Red wine is recommended every day!

The reason this diet pairs well with intermittent fasting is because it contains many of the anti-inflammatory foods that we spoke about earlier and is also one of the least restrictive ways of eating, allowing for socializing with ease. The Mediterranean diet also happens to be the subject of the most scientific studies linking it to improved health, better mood, and longer life.

Ketogenic and Low-Carbohydrate Plans
The ketogenic diet and other lower-carbohydrate plans pair well with intermittent fasting for a number of reasons. First of all, the point of both IF and the keto diet is to direct the body to use stored fat for fuel. Low-carbohydrate diets give your body less glucose to process. When your body is transitioning to ketosis, all of that stored glycogen in your liver and muscles gets used up

and your body starts producing ketones for fuel. Ketones are shown to have an appetite-suppressing effect on the body, making fasting for longer periods easier.

What Not to Eat

That sounds a little harsh to my sensitive ears, especially because I do not believe in villainizing any kind of food. Food is food. Getting wrapped up in calling food "good" or "bad" is pointless and worse, especially when judging what other people are eating. When we judge ourselves by what we put in our own mouths, we put ourselves at risk for disordered eating, orthorexia, and eating disorders. No, thank you! The support groups that I am a part of have a "mind your own plate" policy.

That said, there are foods known to be pro-inflammatory and/or devoid of helpful nutrients but loaded with calories. These kinds of foods should be drastically limited, if not eliminated, when you are putting yourself on a path to greater health with intermittent fasting.

Foods to Avoid

Refined Sugar and High-Fructose Corn Syrup (HFCS) — Sugar and HFCS raise blood glucose levels, which can lead to a spike in inflammation. This effect is more pronounced in people who have any form of glucose intolerance, such as diabetes or insulin resistance.

Soda and Sweetened Soft Drinks — Soda and sweetened drinks are empty calories, have zero health benefit apart from the very short-term mood and energy boosts, and enter the bloodstream quickly due to their liquid form. Many also contain sodium benzoate, a preservative that has been linked to impaired motor function and increased anxiety.

Juice — It is worth mentioning juice here, too. Juice is hailed as a healthy drink, but it is generally high in sugar and stripped of the fiber and many of the nutrients that whole fruits and vegetables contain. The popular chain Jamba Juice has some of the highest calorie drinks in the entire United States! Read labels and nutrition facts so that you know exactly what you are putting in your body.

Artificially Sweetened Beverages — These may have zero calories but create a similar insulin spike to regularly sweetened drinks and they may make you hungrier because of the corresponding blood sugar drop. They are also made with chemicals that the body cannot process that are then stored in fat cells with added water to dilute them. It's worth being mindful of how many you consume and try to opt for water, seltzer, homemade iced teas, and infused waters instead.

Refined Carbohydrates — Think industrially processed bread, pastries, cakes, and pies. Refined carbohydrates have been stripped of their fiber content and are quickly converted to sugar in the body. Many of them also include more sugar and trans fats, two more of the items on this list. Read nutrition and ingredients labels to know what you're eating. Look at the sugar and carb counts in comparison to how much fiber is included. It's better to look for whole-grain versions, make your own baked goods at home, and/or limit the daylights out of these bad boys.

Note: Regarding the previous three items on the list, higher sugar consumption leads to continued sugar cravings. Many people comment that when they have a sugar-infused food blowout, they face super sugar cravings and crankiness the following day, which can make fasting harder.

Excessive Alcohol — Everybody asks the alcohol question! I have never known of something a larger population of people has such a difficult time letting go of emotionally. Here's the good news: I'm not talking about a glass of wine here, even daily. There appear to be several health-promoting consequences of having one drink per day. Outside of that, alcohol is inflammatory. The more you consume, the more inflammation marker C-reactive protein the body produces. Heavy drinkers are more likely to develop fatty liver and be susceptible to detrimental bacteria traveling from the colon back into the intestines and causing what is called "leaky gut," a condition that can create further systemic inflammation. Alcohol may also stall weight loss if that's what you're going for.

Processed Meats — Sorry, chili cheese dog, charcuterie, and bacon fans. Processed meats are any that have been preserved by smoking, salting, curing, or adding chemical preservatives. This includes that sliced turkey you get from the deli! Processed meats have higher levels of advanced glycation end products (AGEs) that studies show create a serious inflammatory response in the body.

Red Meat (consumed excessively) — This may seem contradictory to some of the recently presented information in this book and I personally consider it an iffy topic, but please do read on. Red meat is loaded with protein and has many beneficial attributes including plenty of micronutrients. It produces significantly less AGEs than processed meat, but it does produce them. Consumption has been linked to inflammatory conditions in certain populations. Traditional anti-inflammatory diets recommend limiting red meat. I recommend choosing organic and/or grass-fed red meats whenever you can as they have more nutrient density and add anti-inflammatory components to every beefy meal. Something as simple as adding a slice of anti-inflammatory avocado to your burger—or guacamole to your taco—can offset the inflammatory effects tremendously.

Artificial Trans Fats — Artificial trans fats supplied by margarine and shortening are pretty much the unhealthiest thing you can eat. They're proven to increase inflammation, lower "good" cholesterol, and increase heart disease risks in both men and women. This is why it's a good idea to avoid or limit fried foods, certain margarines and shortenings, mass-produced packaged baked goods, and anything that lists "partially hydrogenated oil" on the label.

Vegetable and Seed Oils — Although we need omega-6 fatty acids in our diets, too many of them (in relation to omega-3s) are highly inflammatory, at least in rat studies. Vegetable and seed oils contain many of them. More research is needed, but it's better to choose unrefined olive and coconut oils when you can.

Foods That Cause Sensitivities and Allergic Reactions — This should seem like a no-brainer, but as a special diet chef and nutritional healing facilitator, I am particularly attuned to seeing people eat foods that make them feel bad and become inflamed just to make life "easier" for the people around them. Allergic reactions are histamine reactions that cause inflammation. Intolerance reactions can cause very uncomfortable inflammation, as well. Avoid foods that make you inflamed, whether it results in visible changes to your skin or belly bloating.

Does this list mean that you need to cut these foods out of your life completely? With the exception of foods that you're allergic to, no. Life is meant for living, and an occasional hot dog, garlic fries, and a soda at the baseball game may be exactly what you want in your eating window—that is 100 percent A-Okay! (I am not giving up bacon or burgers, either.) Use these guidelines, enjoy what you like in moderation, and incorporate more whole, anti-inflammatory foods into your meals every single day.

CHAPTER SEVEN

Fast-Friendly Foods and Drinks

We've just discussed the best foods to eat and avoid during your feasting times. Now what about during your *fasting* times? As fasting is all about not eating and not activating your digestive system, there really are not any foods allowed on a true, clean fast. If you're eating, you're not fasting.

However, if you are fasting for nothing but weight loss, consuming up to 500 calories per day as one would do following the protocol of many popular ADF plans does often still provide the desired benefits and may help with compliance.

This comes with a warning that long-term, consecutive days of consuming 500 or fewer calories amounts to extreme calorie restriction. That is *not* what we're talking about in this book. Long-term calorie restriction has been shown to result in negative metabolic adaptation, a lowered basal metabolic rate (BMR), and weight gain when you transition back to regular eating. Extreme and continuous caloric restriction also makes potential life-threatening micronutrient deficiencies a possibility that cannot be mitigated with a multivitamin. Short-term rapid weight loss may also be accompanied by the loss of hair and lean muscle mass and may negatively affect mental and emotional health.

With this in mind, use the recommendations and food lists that follow to help you get through adaptation to intermittent fasting and/or adjusting to longer fasts. Once you are adapted, you will probably find it even easier to *not* eat at all on fasting days, thereby not hormonally triggering more hunger.

No- and Low-Calorie Foods

Spoiler Alert: There are *no* zero-calorie or reverse-calorie foods, no matter what you've read. The body *always* absorbs some of what you eat, but you can certainly make the most of the volume in ultra-low-calorie foods (usually fruits and vegetables) that make you feel full longer.

The lowest calorie foods per (approximately 1 cup or 100 g) serving include:

- Apples
- Arugula
- Asparagus
- Beets
- Broccoli
- Broth
- Brussels sprouts
- Cabbage
- Carrots
- Cauliflower
- Chard
- Clementines/mandarins
- Cucumbers (and pickles!)
- Fennel
- Fresh herbs
- Grapefruit
- Green beans
- Jicama
- Kale
- Kohlrabi
- Leafy greens in general
- Lemons and limes
- Lettuce
- Mushrooms
- Onions
- Peppers
- Potatoes
- Papaya
- Radishes
- Raspberries
- Rutabaga
- Shirataki noodles and "rice"
- Snow peas
- Spinach
- Strawberries
- Sugar snap peas
- Tomatoes
- Turnips
- Watercress
- Watermelon
- Zucchini

I'll bet you're not surprised that pretty much the entire list consists of fruits and vegetables, and mostly low-carbohydrate ones to boot! You can definitely find ways to fill up on fewer than 500 calories, especially if you mix and match.

No- and Low-Calorie Drinks

There are drinks you can enjoy that will not break a fast and may help fill you up, suppress appetite, and possibly even increase autophagy.

These include:

- Black coffee
- Unsweetened black, green, and white tea
- Unsweetened leaf-based herbal teas (no fruit)
- Plain water
- Water infused (not blended) with fresh herbs, lemon/lime, ginger, turmeric, cinnamon
- Sparkling water (no flavor added)
- Mineral water
- Small amounts of apple cider vinegar (best added to water)

Protein-Sparing Foods

The following is a food list to accompany the traditional Protein Sparing Modified Fast (PSMF) diet that we discussed in chapter 2 (page 19). Everything included is low in carbohydrates and fat and high in protein.

- White meat poultry, preferably chicken breast, turkey, or duck without the skin.
- Low-fat dairy, such as cottage cheese, curd, and skim milk. Ideally, you want to eat the 0 percent fat or 2 percent fat products. Avoid higher fat and flavored cottage cheese.
- Lean white fish such as cod, snapper, grouper, mahi-mahi, ling, sole, halibut, and pike. These fish are significantly milder in flavor and lower in omega-3 fatty acids we associate with salmon, trout, and mackerel.
- Egg whites.
- Tofu, tempeh, and other meat substitutes.
- Lean red meat and organ meats such as heart, liver, and kidneys. Organ meats are particularly nutrient dense.
- Low-carbohydrate vegetables and salad, such as iceberg lettuce, kale, cabbage, spinach, arugula, alfalfa, brassicas, and so on.

Dietary supplements to avoid nutrient deficiencies are part of a standard PSMF plan. Your doctor will be able to advise you, as PSMF is not recommended without medical supervision. Highly bioavailable multivitamins are imperative. Magnesium, iodine, and vitamin D3 are also recommended to ensure your body stays in working order.

The following are not recommended on a PSMF:

- Liquid calories, unless they are in soup (They will not fill you up and likely contain higher carbohydrates than is recommended.)
- Any high-carb foods and/or starches
- Added fat of any type

CHAPTER EIGHT

Meal Planning

You now know what your body needs, the best foods to eat to achieve that, and which foods to avoid (or limit) to make this intermittent fasting journey a pleasant and successful one. It's time to figure out how to actually feed yourself during your feasting times to make the most of them and stay on track as much as possible! Meal planning is one of the best accountability tools out there to do just that.

There are countless free and for-purchase meal plans online and a growing number of apps to help you make it happen. The best way to ensure that you are getting the nutrients you need through food that you actually want to eat is to plan meals for yourself.

As a chef, I plan meals for my delivery clients every week for the following week. Designing a menu in advance helps me figure out exactly what I need to buy at the store and what I already have on hand, saving both money and time.

I also meal plan for myself using the same principles, and it makes life so much easier when my feasting window opens, *especially* when I combine it with meal prep. Having the ingredients I need on hand—already chopped, marinated, or cooked—makes it much more likely that I will get the nutrients I want in a healthy form as opposed to a mish-mash of macros that doesn't quite fit the bill.

How to Meal Plan

Once you have decided which fasting schedule you are going to follow and what your caloric needs are, it's time to choose how many meals you need to plan and for how many days. This may be defined by something as simple as how frequently you aim to grocery shop during the week.

You also want to factor in whether you will be dining out and not plan to cook for those days. To stay on track during restaurant days, it's a good idea to go online and choose what you might like from the menu before you get there—hungry can mean having a hard time making decisions.

Next, decide which kind of foods you want to eat and do some research! Spend time browsing through cookbooks, magazines, blogs, and Pinterest to find dishes that turn up your interest. Create a place to save the recipes you want to try, whether online or in a notebook. Of course, I recommend that you choose nutrient-dense ones loaded with all of the yummy ingredients that you read about earlier, but if you feel like fettuccine Alfredo one night, plan it! Make a note of the calorie count to ensure that it fits in your day, especially as you are getting used to IF.

For ADF practitioners, it is a great idea to find multiple low-calorie-per-serving recipes so that you can create multiple small meals in a day. It's also fine to have multiple servings at one time to have one bulkier meal and cook less!

Another cooking-less tip is to seek out recipes that you can pre-portion and enjoy multiple times in a week. Casseroles are great for this. Rotisserie chickens can be transformed into all sorts of dishes and are one of my personal go-to picks to cook as little as possible outside of what I do for work.

I also like to read circulars and check what's on sale. That may shape which recipes I decide to try in a given week *and* save me a few bucks while I'm at it.

At this point, it's time to write down the ingredients you need and make your shopping list. Take an inventory of what you already have in your pantry, fridge, and freezer and cross those off the list before you go shopping so you don't buy doubles. I once found myself with four cans of baking powder from different shopping trips. It eventually all got used, but it was a little crazy to realize I had so much on hand.

Speaking of which, make sure you always have your staples on hand, such as olive oil, your go-to spices, and whatever canned goods you use frequently. For me, that means always having cans of tuna, sardines, coconut milk, chicken broth, and diced tomatoes.

Take a look at your calendar and decide which day looks best for shopping and prepping. I usually shop the grocery store on Friday and the farmers' market on Saturday, and meal prep on Sunday, but it's whatever works best for your schedule. Weekend days tend to be the busiest time at the shops, so it will usually take longer.

List in hand, go shopping. Sticking to the list will save you both money and time.

If you CAN, shop and prep the same day. You don't have to prepare all your meals in their entirety, but roasting a bunch of chicken thighs while pre-chopping the vegetables you plan to use during the week will make meals come together much more quickly when you need them to.

It's worth considering signing up for meal plans through an app (see Useful Apps, page 187) that will automatically generate your shopping list for you. You can also do a Google or Pinterest search for a meal plan featuring almost any kind of dietary requirement, and I guarantee multiple plans will show up, some with grocery lists already included.

If you hate shopping more than anything and can afford the cost, meal kits from companies such as Sun Basket, Blue Apron, Hello Fresh, Green Chef, Purple Carrot, and more can simplify your life tremendously. With Freshly, you don't even have to cook—you just have to reheat. (I am not endorsing any particular companies here. I'm just trying to be real and acknowledge that not everybody loves reading recipes and roaming the aisles of the grocery store as much as I do.)

3

The Recipes

"One cannot think well, love well, sleep well,
if one has not dined well."

—VIRGINIA WOOLF

Let's get cooking! Every single one of the recipes that follow
was crafted with "dining well" in mind. By dining well, I
mean dining for wellness, dining to flood your body with
micronutrients while causing your taste buds to do a happy
dance, dining to fuel your cells *and* your soul. Healthy and
delicious are not meant to be mutually exclusive. So treat
yourself—and your friends and family, too—by enjoying all the
yumminess in the pages ahead!

CHAPTER NINE

Let's Get Cooking! Nutrient-Dense Recipes to Feast Upon

Filling Snacks

Snacks are a smart and strategic way to squeeze extra nutrients into your day and also help keep you from overeating when it comes to the "big" mealtimes! Choosing healthy, balanced, and nutrient-dense options will keep your blood sugar steady and your fasting plan on track!

I like to keep a batch of most of these recipes on hand for when hunger arrives out of the blue or when my feasting window opens but I haven't figured out what I want to eat for my meal yet. High-Protein Vegan Crackers (page 59) or chopped fresh vegetables dipped in Sunflower Seed Muhammara (page 61) or Low-Carb Spiced Cauliflower Hummus (page 62) are heavenly ways to calm your cravings while getting so many nutrients in—and they are perfect to share with friends, too!

High-Protein Vegan Crackers

These crackers are cakey without being crumbly, and they're just begging to be topped with cheese and meats or dipped into something luscious. At only 4 grams of net carbs, 13 grams of protein, and 14 grams of fat per serving, these plant-based crackers are guaranteed to satisfy.

Total time: 50 minutes   **Yield:** 48 crackers

½ cup (120 ml) water

3 tablespoons (21 g) flaxseed meal

½ cup (80 g) unflavored hemp protein

½ cup (52 g) almond flour

¼ cup (28 g) coconut flour

3 tablespoons (21 g) hemp hearts or sesame seeds

1 tablespoon (11 g) chia seeds

¼ teaspoon fine salt, preferably Himalayan

1 tablespoon (14 g) coconut oil, melted

Optional seasonings:

¼ teaspoon garlic powder, paprika, rosemary, herbs de Provence, chili powder, cumin, or caraway seed

Accessories needed:

Parchment paper

Baking tray

Mixing bowls

Rolling pin

Preheat the oven to 350°F (175°C, or gas mark 4) with a rack placed in the middle. Prepare a piece of parchment paper twice as long as the baking tray you will be using. You will be folding it over to roll out the crackers and half will be discarded at the time of cooking.

In a small bowl, whisk together the water and flaxseed meal. Set aside. In a medium bowl, stir together all the dry ingredients (including any seasonings, if using) with a fork until well blended. Add the flax-water mixture and coconut oil and stir well, forming into a ball. It should be pliable and not crumbly.

Set the parchment paper on a flat surface and place the dough near the center. Fold the paper upward until the edges meet. You can do this on your baking tray if your rolling tool is narrow enough—a large bottle will work in a pinch. Press down on the dough ball to flatten slightly and then roll it out to a 9- x 12-inch (23 x 30 cm) rectangle about ⅛ inch (3 mm) thick. Cut off the top layer of the paper.

Use a knife or pizza cutter to cut the dough into six strips and then eight crackers per strip.

Bake for 30 minutes. Remove the tray, flip the crackers, and return to the oven for 10 minutes. Remove and allow to cool completely.

These keep for 10 days in the pantry, no refrigeration needed.

Nutritional Information (8 crackers): Calories: 193 – Protein: 13 g – Fat: 14 g – Carbs: 7.5 g – Fiber: 3.5 g – Net carbs: 4 g – Sodium: 178 mg – Potassium: 238 mg

Sunflower Seed Muhammara

Muhammara is a richly flavored Middle Eastern dipping sauce traditionally made with walnuts, roasted red peppers, spicy red chili, and pomegranate molasses. To create a delicious and milder version that would appeal to even those with nut allergies, I swapped in sunflower seeds and BOY was that a great idea! The texture is the same, the flavor profile is a little bit brighter, and the nutrient density is heartily increased as sunflower seeds far outshine walnuts in potassium, iron, magnesium, and vitamin B_6 gram for gram.

Total time: 5 minutes   **Yield:** 8 servings

¾ cup (110 g) toasted sunflower seeds

¼ cup (60 ml) extra virgin olive oil

1½ tablespoons (22 ml) pomegranate molasses*, yacon syrup*, or both
(I used 1 tablespoon yacon + ½ tablespoon pomegranate molasses)

1 teaspoon sweet smoked paprika

Pinch cayenne pepper or red pepper flakes*

½ teaspoon cumin

½ teaspoon salt

One 7-ounce (210 ml) jar roasted peppers

Accessory needed:

Food processor or high-speed blender

Combine all ingredients in a food processor or high-speed blender until smooth. Enjoy with raw vegetables, crackers, breads, or whatever you like! This dipping sauce keeps 3 days in an airtight container in the refrigerator.

Nutritional Information: Calories: 150 – Protein: 2.6 g – Fat: 14 g – Carbs: 6.4 g – Fiber: 1.5 g – Net carbs: 4.9 g – Sodium: 868 mg – Potassium: 176 mg

Note:

Pomegranate molasses, a thick pomegranate syrup, can be found at Middle Eastern markets, some supermarkets, and online. Yacon syrup can usually be found at health food stores and online. To make the most authentic and spicy version of this dipping sauce, look for Aleppo pepper paste or flakes.

Low-Carb Spiced Cauliflower Hummus

Enjoy the deliciousness of hummus while getting an extra serving of vegetables!
This low-carb version of everybody's favorite dip tastes so similar to the original, your friends and family may not even notice that there is not a chickpea in sight. Pro-tip: This recipe is a perfect accompaniment for the Broccoli-Hemp Heart Falafel (page 170), providing a double dose of sulforaphane with the classic mild flavor of traditional hummus.

Total time: 35 minutes   **Yield:** 8 servings

1 pound (455 g) cauliflower florets, torn into bite-size pieces

2 tablespoons (30 ml) extra-virgin olive oil

1 teaspoon ground cumin

½ teaspoon ground coriander

½ teaspoon smoked paprika

½ teaspoon salt, plus more to taste

⅓ cup (80 ml) tahini

Zest and juice of 1 lemon

2 teaspoons (6 g) minced garlic

¼–½ cup (60–120 ml) water

1 teaspoon sesame oil, plus more to taste

Olive oil (optional)

Accessories needed:

Baking tray

Parchment paper

Food processor or blender

Preheat the oven to 400°F (200°C, or gas mark 6). Line the baking tray with parchment paper and place the cauliflower on top. Drizzle olive oil over the cauliflower and sprinkle with the cumin, coriander, paprika, and salt. Toss until the pieces are evenly coated. Bake for 25 minutes.

Transfer the cauliflower to a food processor or blender and add the tahini, lemon zest and juice, garlic, and ¼ cup (60 ml) water. Process or blend until smooth. You may have to scrape down the sides of the bowl a couple of times to get the right consistency. Add more water, 1 tablespoon (15 ml) at a time, for a thinner consistency. Transfer to a serving dish and stir in the sesame oil. Drizzle with additional sesame or olive oil (if using), as desired. Enjoy!

Nutritional Information (¼ cup): Calories: 112 – Protein: 3 g – Fat: 9.5 g – Carbs: 5.8 g – Fiber: 1.8 g – Net carbs: 4 g – Sodium: 197 mg – Potassium: 233 mg

Everyman Tzatziki

This tzatziki is creamy, crunchy, herby, citrusy, and perfect for dipping and slathering on fish, chicken, and lamb. This cucumber yumminess is super customizable to your dietary requirements. I love anything and everything full fat, but you can also use fat-free yogurt for calorie minimization.

Prep time: 5 minutes **Cook Time:** N/A **Serves:** 2 cups

1 cup (230 g) yogurt, crème fraîche, or dairy-free yogurt alternative, such as Coyo

½ cup (70 g) finely chopped cucumber

1 green onion, finely chopped

1 clove garlic, minced

1 tablespoon (6 g) finely chopped fresh mint

1 tablespoon (4 g) finely chopped fresh dill

Juice and zest of ½ a lemon (1–2 tablespoons)

⅛ - ¼ teaspoon salt

Accessory needed:

Mixing bowl

Combine all the ingredients in a small mixing bowl. The tzatziki will last for 3 days in an airtight container in the fridge.

Nutritional Information (based on fattiest crème fraîche): Calories: 103 – Protein: 1 g – Fat: 10 g – Carbs: 1.75 g – Fiber: .75 g – Net carbs: 1 g – Sodium: 80 mg – Potassium: 7.5 mg

Low-Carb Peanut Butter Cookies

Sometimes, you just need a cookie. Especially one that marries peanut butter and chocolate! These high-fat, high-protein, low-sugar cookies are a delightful sweet treat to crush your sweet craving without giving you a sugar crash later.

Total time: 30 minutes   **Yield:** 16 cookies

1 cup (260 g) no-sugar-added crunchy peanut butter

1 egg, beaten lightly

¼ cup (60 g) stevia-sweetened or ultra-dark chocolate chips

¼ cup (60 ml) erythritol syrup (such as Sukrin Gold fiber syrup), yacon syrup, or honey (if you're okay with a higher carbohydrate option)

1 teaspoon baking soda

Accessories needed:

Baking tray

Parchment paper

Mixing bowl

Preheat the oven to 375°F (190°C, or gas mark 5). Line a baking tray with parchment paper.

Combine all the ingredients in the mixing bowl and drop by the tablespoonful onto the tray about 2 inches (5 cm) apart until the mixture is finished.

Bake for 10 minutes. Cool for 10 minutes on the baking tray; they will be too soft while warm to transfer anywhere else (apart from your mouth!).

Nutritional Information (1 cookie): Calories: 132 – Protein: 4.7 g – Fat: 9.6 g – Carbs: 8.7 g – Fiber: 1.6 g – Net carbs: 7.1 g – Sodium: 146 mg – Potassium: 127 mg

Sweet and Salty Spiced Almonds

One handful of these nuts, whether you make them sugary or sugar-free, will quell the hungries in no time flat with their well-balanced protein, fat, and fiber ratios. They are the perfect portable snack to carry around, especially when you want to open your feasting window but aren't yet ready for a full meal.

Total time: 45 minutes   **Yield:** 8 servings

1 egg white

2 cups (290 g) raw almonds

¼ cup (50 g) fine granulated sugar or sugar substitute, such as monk fruit (see note)

2 teaspoons (4 g) garam masala or ras el hanout spice blend

½ teaspoon fine Himalayan salt

Accessories needed:

Baking tray

Parchment paper

Mixing bowls

Preheat the oven to 350°F (175°C, or gas mark 4). Line a baking tray with parchment paper.

In a medium bowl, whisk the egg white until frothy. Add the almonds and combine.

In a separate small bowl, combine the sugar, garam masala, and salt. Pour the dry ingredients in the almond mixture and toss until all are well coated.

Transfer to the lined baking tray and bake for 20 minutes. Remove from the oven, stir the almonds, and return to the oven for 10 minutes. Cool completely.

Enjoy immediately or store for up to 3 days at room temperature.

Nutritional Information (using sugar): Calories: 186 – Protein: 6.3 g – Fat: 14 g – Carbs: 12 g – Fiber: 3.5 g – Net carbs: 8.5 g – Sodium: 170 mg – Potassium: 211 mg

Notes

Monk fruit will be significantly darker than regular sugar when baked.

Dark Chocolate Almond Power Balls

Sometimes when your eating window is opening or coming to a close, you might need just one little bite of something to soothe the savage beast in your belly! For me, it's usually when I'm opening my feasting window and have yet to decide what to eat. To ensure that my eyes accurately reflect the size of my stomach, I keep these ultra-satisfying and tasty little guys on hand. They include chocolate, but they're more of a savory snack loaded with beneficial polyphenols, vitamins, minerals, and healthy fats.

Total time: 40 minutes (including chilling time)   **Yield:** about 24 pieces, 3 pieces per serving

1 cup (110 g) shaved almonds

1 cup (260 g) almond butter

½ cup (70 g) pumpkin seeds

⅓ cup (59 g) chia seeds

¼ cup (36 g) sunflower seeds

¼ cup (21 g) unsweetened flaked coconut

2 tablespoons (10 g) cocoa powder, divided

1 teaspoon vanilla extract

½ teaspoon fine salt

Accessories needed:

Food processor

Baking tray

Parchment paper

2-tablespoon (30 ml) portion scoop

Pie pan or small bowl

Combine all the ingredients, except for 1 tablespoon (5 g) cocoa powder, in the food processor and pulse until a mostly smooth paste is formed. I like the texture of slightly larger almond and pumpkin seed pieces to make this high-protein, high-fat snack feel even more filling!

Line a baking tray with parchment paper. Scoop the mixture into 2-tablespoon portions and place on the baking tray. Place the remaining tablespoon of cocoa powder into the pie plate or bowl. Moisten your hands slightly, roll each mound between your palms into a smooth ball, and then roll in the extra cocoa powder to coat. Place back on the parchment-lined tray. Transfer to the freezer to chill and firm up for 30 minutes. Store these in an airtight container in the refrigerator for up to 3 weeks.

Nutritional Information (using sugar): Calories: 320 – Protein: 11 g – Fat: 27 g – Carbs: 14 g – Fiber: 7.7 g – Net carbs: 6.3 g – Sodium: 371 mg – Potassium: 382 mg

Breakfast

Are you a morning person? I certainly am. And that makes breakfast (and all breakfast foods!) among my most preferred— at ANY time of day! Just about all of these recipes can be made ahead in batches for you to grab-and-go and enjoy throughout the week.

Try making a fruit and yogurt parfait with a layer of protein-rich No Grainola (page 74). Give yourself a chocolate moustache with a fantastically filling and incredibly tasty Chococado Coconut Smoothie (page 80). Or make your eggs for the whole week with a batch of one of my client favorites, Broccoli and Caramelized Onion Egg Bites (page 81)!

Break-Fast Bibimbap with Sesame Fried Egg

Bibimbap is one of my favorite dishes. It looks complicated, but it comes together quickly once the chopping is done, and you can shortcut most of the recipe with precut veggies from the grocery store. It's ultra-high in a variety of nutrients, and the kimchi gives you a great dose of probiotics, as well. Although I prefer mine with either shirataki or cauliflower rice to keep it low carb, traditional rice is a delicious addition, whether you choose white, brown, red, forbidden, or something else. Substitute away!

Total time: 30 minutes   **Yield:** 2 servings

4 cups (940 ml) water

Salt

1 medium carrot, julienned

1 cup (71 g) broccoli florets, broken into bite-size or smaller pieces

1 cup (50 g) mung bean sprouts

4 teaspoons (20 ml) sesame oil, divided

1 packet (8 ounces, or 225 g) rinsed and drained shirataki rice (such as Miracle Rice), 1 cup (113 g) cauliflower rice, or 1 cup (186 g) steamed white rice (note calorie/carb differences)

2 eggs

¼ cup (60 g) prepared kimchi

¼ cup (2 g) shredded toasted nori (optional)

1 tablespoon (8 g) toasted sesame seeds

Gochujang Korean hot sauce or crushed red pepper flakes (optional)

Accessories needed:

2-quart (2 L) saucepan

Slotted spoon

Small mixing bowls

Small frying pan

Bring the water and ½ teaspoon salt to a boil in the saucepan over medium-high heat. Add the carrots and blanch for 30 seconds, until they are just becoming flexible. Remove with a slotted spoon and set aside on a plate or in a small bowl. Repeat the process with the broccoli and bean sprouts. Drizzle each vegetable with ½ teaspoon of sesame oil and with salt to taste.

Heat the small frying pan over medium-high heat until a drop of water sizzles upon contact.

If using shirataki rice, be sure to drain the packet and rinse before adding to the hot pan to dry fry. Allow the moisture to cook out and the rice to turn opaque, stirring frequently. Remove from the pan and set aside.

Break-Fast Bibimbap with Sesame Fried Egg
(continued from page 71)

If using cauliflower rice, combine 3 tablespoons (45 ml) of water and 1 cup (113 g) of cauliflower rice and add to the frying pan, stirring until all the liquid has evaporated. Remove from the pan and set aside.

Crack the two eggs into a small bowl, being careful not to break the yolks.

Rinse the saucepan and replace on the stove over medium-high heat until a drop of water sizzles upon contact again. Add the remaining sesame oil. Once it runs freely around the pan, lower the heat to medium and gently pour the eggs into the pan, separating them by drawing a line between them with a spatula. Sprinkle each with a pinch of salt. Cook, uncovered, for about 4 minutes, allowing the bottoms to brown and become slightly crispy by the time the tops of the whites are set. For less crispy eggs, turn the heat to low instead and cook, covered, for 2 to 2½ minutes.

Turn off heat and start building your bowls. Bibimbap traditionally gets all mixed up when you start eating it but is super photo-worthy before that first bite! Divide the rice into two bowls. For each bowl, arrange half of the toppings in individual little piles on top of the rice, working in a clockwise fashion with the broccoli, carrots, bean sprouts, kimchi, and nori shreds (if using). Lay the egg on top and sprinkle each bowl with ½ tablespoon sesame seeds. Drizzle with gochujang, if desired, to make it extra spicy.

When you eat it, make sure to tear into that runny egg yolk to give your bowl some extra sauciness!

Nutritional Information: Calories: 236 – Protein: 12g – Fat: 16.5 g – Carbs: 14 g – Fiber: 4.8 g – Net carbs: 9.2 g – Sodium: 771 mg – Potassium: 615 mg

No Grainola

I love the *idea* of granola, with its crispy-crunchy, slightly sweet, slightly salty goodness that's perfect for enjoying by the handful, in almond milk, or as a layer in a perfect parfait. But I *don't* like the low nutrient density and carbs that come along with most commercially prepared ones. Enter this grain-free, Paleo- and keto-friendly version that tastes a little like a sweet and salty pretzel!

Total time: 40 minutes (including cooling time)   **Yield:** 20 servings

1 egg white

¼ cup (60 ml) extra-virgin olive oil

2 tablespoons (30 ml) maple syrup, yacon syrup, or maple-flavored monk fruit syrup

1 teaspoon ground cinnamon

1 teaspoon vanilla powder

½ teaspoon fine salt

2 cups (220 g) shaved almonds

½ cup (68 g) chopped raw cashews

½ cup (55 g) chopped raw pecans

½ cup (60 g) hemp hearts

½ cup (88 g) chia seeds

½ cup (70 g) raw pumpkin seeds

½ cup (42 g) unsweetened flaked coconut

Accessories needed:

Baking tray

Parchment paper

Mixing bowls

Preheat the oven 350°F (175°C, or gas mark 4). Line a standard baking tray with parchment paper.

In a large mixing bowl, whisk together the egg white, olive oil, syrup, cinnamon, vanilla, and salt until frothy and partially emulsified. Add all the nuts and seeds and toss well to coat.

Spread on the baking tray in a single layer. Bake for 25 minutes. Remove from the oven and cool for at least 10 minutes before enjoying. Store this yummy blend in an airtight container for up to 1 week, in the fridge for 2 weeks, or in the freezer for up to 2 months.

Nutritional Information (about ¼ cup [30 g]): Calories: 212 – Protein: 6.3 g – Fat: 18 g – Carbs: 10 g – Fiber: 4.2 g – Net carbs: 5.8 g – Sodium: 132 mg – Potassium: 228 mg

Bacon, Basil, and Tomato Quiche-Lettes

Oh, summery tasting egg muffins, how do I love thee? These quick, crustless quiche muffins have the flavors of a BLT, are a worthy addition to your weekly meal prep—and they freeze and travel well. There is no excuse to let that ultra-nutritious extra summer basil go to waste ever again!

Total time: 34 minutes   **Yield:** 4 servings (3 pieces)

---

1 cup (8 ounces) cooked bacon, crumbled

½ cup (80 g) chopped red onion

½ cup (30 g) tightly packed fresh basil

½ cup (62 g) chopped grape or cherry tomatoes

3 tablespoons (21 g) coconut flour

6 eggs

Pinch of salt and black pepper

Olive or avocado cooking spray, 1 tablespoon (15 ml) oil, or 1 tablespoon (15 ml) bacon grease

Accessories needed:

Mixing bowl

12-well muffin pan

Preheat the oven to 350°F (175°C, or gas mark 4).

Combine all the ingredients except the cooking spray in a mixing bowl and whisk together. Set aside for 5 minutes to allow to thicken slightly.

Grease the muffin tin with the cooking spray. Divide the muffin mixture evenly among the twelve wells in the muffin pan.

Bake for 19 minutes. Remove from the oven and cool for 5 minutes. Slide a butter knife around the edge of the muffin wells to remove the muffins.

Enjoy immediately or refrigerate in an airtight container for up to 4 days. Freeze for up to 2 months, reheating in the microwave for 2 minutes.

Nutritional Information: Calories: 261 - Protein: 18.5 g - Fat: 16.25 g - Carbs: 5.75 g - Fiber: 2.75 g - Net carbs: 3 g - Sodium: 618 mg - Potassium: 104 mg

Hemp Heart Porridge with Apples and Cinnamon

Remember those powdery packets of apple cinnamon oatmeal that you thought were the most delicious thing ever? Well, this is the grown-up version—low in carbs, high in protein, and bursting with nutrients.

Total time: 10 minutes   **Yield:** 2 servings

1 cup (240 ml) unsweetened hemp or almond milk

½ teaspoon vanilla powder

Pinch of Himalayan salt

½ teaspoon ground cinnamon

½ cup (60 g) hemp hearts

½ cup (63 g) flaxseed meal

½ cup (55 g) grated, unpeeled apple plus extra for topping

2 teaspoons (10 ml) MCT oil, such as Nutiva, NOW Foods, Bulletproof Brain Octane (optional)

Chopped toasted walnuts (optional)

½ teaspoon brown sugar or brown sugar substitute, such as Sukrin, coconut sugar, or maple sugar

Accessory needed:

Small saucepan

Heat the milk over medium-high heat and whisk in the vanilla powder, salt, and cinnamon. At the first sign of a boil, whisk in the hemp hearts and flaxseed meal. Lower the heat to medium and stir. As the mixture thickens, stir in the apple.

Once it looks like all liquid has been absorbed, remove from the heat and stir in the MCT oil (if using). Transfer to serving bowls. Garnish with extra grated apple, toasted walnuts (if using), and brown sugar.

Nutritional Information (with MCT oil): Calories: 462 – Protein: 20 g – Fat: 35 g – Carbs: 20 g – Fiber: 13.5 g – Net carbs: 6.5 g – Sodium: 80 mg – Potassium: 288 mg

Golden Milk Chia Pudding

This recipe has all the good, anti-inflammatory benefits of turmeric-infused golden milk in a happy little chia pudding!

Total time: 15 minutes (including setting time) **Yield:** 2 servings

---

½ cup (88 g) chia seeds

½ teaspoon turmeric

¼ teaspoon ground cinnamon

¼ teaspoon vanilla powder or extract

¼ teaspoon ground ginger

¼ teaspoon ground cardamom

Pinch of Himalayan salt

Pinch of ground black pepper

1 cup (240 ml) unsweetened nut-based, hemp, or other plant-based milk

½ cup (120 ml) full-fat coconut milk

Liquid stevia or monk fruit

Accessory needed:

Small mixing bowl

Add all the ingredients from the chia seeds through to the black pepper to a small mixing bowl and combine well. Whisk in the nut milk, coconut milk, and 4 to 5 drops of liquid sweetener. Let sit for 10 to 15 minutes to thicken. Taste and adjust the flavor with more sweetener if necessary.

Nutritional Information (using almond milk): Calories: 354 – Protein: 12.5 g – Fat: 23 g – Carbs: 23 g – Fiber: 20.5 g – Net carbs: 2.5 g – Sodium: 151 mg – Potassium: 256 mg

Chococado Coconut Smoothie

Decadent and delicious, this smoothie is super thick, creamy, and satisfies while providing plenty of healthy fats, heaps of magnesium, and quite the tasty supply of potassium, too! Although the recipe is only for one serving, you can easily double, triple, or quadruple it and store it pre-portioned in the fridge for a few days. The only trouble is limiting yourself to just one.

Total time: 5 minutes   **Yield:** 1 serving

½ cup (120 ml) full-fat coconut milk

½ of a medium avocado, peeled and pitted

1 tablespoon (6 g) cacao powder

10 drops stevia

¼ teaspoon vanilla extract

½ cup (120 ml) almond milk

A few ice cubes

⅛ teaspoon salt

Accessory needed:

Blender

Combine all the ingredients in a blender and blend until smooth. Enjoy immediately or store in an airtight container in the refrigerator for 3 to 4 days.

Nutritional Information: Calories: 341 – Protein: 5 g – Fat: 31 g – Carbs: 13 g – Fiber: 7 g – Net carbs: 6 g – Sodium: 134 mg – Potassium: 595 mg

Broccoli and Caramelized Onion Egg Bites

These delicious little bites can be made in bulk, so you can have them for days!
The serving size is two whole egg bites, but they are so filling, you may have a hard
time getting there. Luckily, they freeze well, too.

Total time: 40 minutes **Yield:** 6 servings (2 egg bites per serving)

2 tablespoons (30 ml)
extra-virgin olive oil, plus more
for greasing

1 cup (115 g) thinly sliced onion

Salt

8 eggs

2 cups (480 g) broccoli
rice (see note)

Pinch of black pepper

Accessories needed:

Small frying pan

Medium mixing bowl

Twelve ½-cup (120-ml)
canning jars with lids

Baking tray

Preheat the oven to 400°F (200°C, or gas mark 6).

Place 2 tablespoons (30 ml) of the olive oil in the frying pan over medium-high heat and warm the oil until it runs around the pan easily. Add the onions and a pinch of salt. Stir frequently for about 10 minutes, making sure the onions soften and start to caramelize but don't burn. Once the onions are soft, remove from the heat and allow to cool for a couple of minutes.

Meanwhile, whisk the eggs and broccoli together with a pinch of salt and pepper. Grease the inside of the jars with olive oil and place on a baking tray.

Stir the onions into the broccoli and egg mixture and divide among the twelve jars. Bake for 15 to 20 minutes, until the tops no longer show any signs of liquid and are springy-firm to the touch. Remove, let cool, and enjoy.

You can also make this recipe using the sous vide method, and it comes out more like a savory broccoli flan. Heat a water bath to 170°F (77°C). Once the egg mixture has been distributed among the jars, attach the lids so they are fingertip tight. That means closed and then turned back a quarter of a turn so that air bubbles can escape. Drop in the bath for 30 to 35 minutes and voilà—they're done!

Nutritional Information: Calories: 155 - Protein: 9.5 g - Fat: 11 g – Carbs: 4.7 g - Fiber: 1.2 g - Net carbs: 3.5 g - Sodium: 106 mg – Potassium: 222 mg

Note:

Riced broccoli is something you may be able to buy at your local grocery store. If not, it can be made using the same techniques as cauliflower rice, either by pulsing in a food processor using the S-blade or grating attachment *or* grating by hand on a box grater using the largest hole.

Keto Matcha Crepes

This recipe is like a matcha latte, but in a crepe! Matcha has been shown to boost energy *and* concentration, provide the same antioxidant benefits as regular green tea, and help boost weight loss—among other pluses. These crepes are delicate in both texture and flavor. To make them a little more pliable, add an extra egg *or* ¼ teaspoon of xanthan gum to the stated recipe.

Total time: 20 minutes   **Yield:** 2 servings (2 crepes per serving)

3 large eggs

½ cup (120 ml) reduced fat coconut, almond, or hemp milk, plus a little more

¼ cup (28 g) coconut flour

1 tablespoon (6 g) matcha powder

5 drops liquid stevia or liquid monk fruit

1 tablespoon (15 ml) avocado oil or ghee

Whipped cream, whipped coconut cream, powdered sugar or sugar substitute

Accessories needed:

Medium mixing bowl

9-inch (23-cm) or smaller nonstick frying pan

Rubber spatula

Break the eggs into the mixing bowl and beat until uniform. Add the milk, coconut flour, matcha, stevia, and whisk until well combined and smooth. The coconut flour will thicken up the mixture. Add 1 to 2 tablespoons (15 to 30 ml) more milk to thin it slightly, if desired.

Heat the frying pan over medium-high heat until a drop of water sizzles on contact. Add the avocado oil and swirl to coat the pan. Add ⅓ cup (80 ml) of the batter to the pan and tilt pan in all directions to spread it into a thin layer. Cook for 1 to 2 minutes until the top looks mostly dry before gently flipping with a rubber spatula. Cook for 20 to 30 seconds and tip over onto a waiting plate. Repeat the process until the batter is gone.

Serve with whipped cream, whipped coconut cream, or a small amount of powdered sugar or sugar substitute. Yum!

Nutritional Information: Calories: 250 – Protein: 11 g – Fat: 17.5 g – Carbs: 11 g – Fiber: 5 g – Net carbs: 6 g – Sodium: 176 mg – Potassium: 0 mg

Soups

Soups are an incredibly healthy addition to your regular meal rotation. They warm your body and mood at the same time, and they've also been proven to be one of the most filling and satisfying food choices on earth! Not only that, soups tend to be extra nutrient dense and contribute to hydration with high liquid content.

Going for an extended fast? Break it gently with Fast-Breaking Vegetable Soup (page 84), a great choice to open your feasting window ANY day, really! Want to take a culinary trip to an Italian home-kitchen without ever leaving your neighborhood? Try the richly flavored and textured, yet simple to make, Italian Sausage Soup (page 87). No matter which option you choose, you will finish your bowl with a happy, nourished belly.

Fast-Breaking Vegetable Soup

Eating this soup is like eating a rainbow because of how colorful it is. It's perfect for breaking an extended fast or enjoying anytime. This simple, light, and nutritious soup is guaranteed to brighten your day.

Total time: 35 minutes   **Yield:** 4 servings

2 tablespoons (30 ml) extra-virgin olive oil

½ cup (65 g) chopped carrot

½ cup (50 g) chopped celery

½ cup (80 g) chopped onion

½ cup (60 g) chopped yellow squash

½ cup (35 g) chopped mushrooms

½ cup (45 g) chopped cabbage

½ cup (50 g) chopped green beans

¼ teaspoon fine salt, plus more to taste

½ teaspoon Italian seasoning

1 can (14.5 ounces, or 411 g) fire-roasted diced tomatoes

2 cups (475 ml) bone broth, such as low-sodium chicken bone broth

Black pepper

Accessory needed:

Medium saucepan

Heat the oil in the saucepan over medium-high heat. Add all the raw vegetables (carrot through green beans), salt, and Italian seasoning. Sauté for 5 minutes, stirring frequently. Add the tomatoes and cook for 5 minutes, allowing some of the liquid to cook off.

Pour in the bone broth. Bring to a rolling boil for 2 minutes before lowering the heat to medium-low and simmering for 5 minutes. Season with salt and pepper and enjoy!

Nutritional Information: Calories: 123 – Protein: 6.8 g – Fat: 7.3 g – Carbs: 9.6 g – Fiber: 3.8 g – Net carbs: 5.8 g – Sodium: 531 mg – Potassium: 429 mg

Italian Sausage Soup

Hearty is the name of the game here. You can make this soup ultra-low-carb by replacing the beans with cauliflower florets. Either way, you're getting a seriously tasty superfood bonanza!

Total time: 35 minutes   **Yield:** 6 servings

2 tablespoons (30 ml) extra-virgin olive oil

1 pound (455 g) hot or mild Italian sausage, bought in bulk or removed from casings

1 cup (100 g) chopped celery

½ cup (80 g) chopped onion

1 teaspoon Italian seasoning

3 cups (705 ml) bone broth, preferably beef, though chicken will work, too

1 can (14.5 ounces, or 411 g) diced tomatoes

1 can (15 ounces, or 425 g) cannellini beans, drained and rinsed (optional)

1 can (15 ounces, or 425 g) kidney beans, drained and rinsed (optional)

1 medium carrot, grated (about ½ cup)

2 cups (200 g) bite-size cauliflower florets, raw (optional)

Salt and black pepper

Accessory needed:

Large saucepan

Add the oil to the saucepan over medium-high heat. Once it runs freely around the pan, crumble in the Italian sausage and add the celery, onion, and Italian seasoning. Stir frequently to prevent the vegetables from burning and break apart the larger pieces of sausage. Cook, for about 5 minutes, until the sausage is cooked through.

Add the bone broth and tomatoes and bring to a light boil for about 5 minutes. Reduce the heat and simmer for 10 minutes. If using cauliflower instead of the beans, add it to the pot for the simmer.

Stir in the beans (if using) and carrots and cook for a final 5 minutes. Season with salt and pepper to taste. Divide among six serving bowls and enjoy!

Nutritional Information (made with beans): Calories: 373 –
Protein: 23 g – Fat: 20.5 g – Carbs: 23.5 g – Fiber: 6.5 g – Net carbs: 17 g –
Sodium: 988 mg – Potassium: 680 mg

Chicken, Rice and Zucchini Soup & Parsley Pistou

With the addition of bright yellow turmeric, plenty of garlic and onions, and a swirl of super-nutritious, cleansing parsley, this is an extra anti-inflammatory twist on homey, yummy chicken and rice soup that you will love no matter the weather outside!

Total time: 25 minutes   **Yield:** 5 servings

2 tablespoons (30 ml) extra-virgin olive oil

1 cup (160 g) chopped onion

½ tablespoon (5 g) minced garlic

1 teaspoon salt

½ teaspoon ground turmeric

4 cups (940 ml) low-sodium bone broth

2 cups (280 g) cooked shredded chicken

1 cup (120 g) chopped or spiralized zucchini

1 packet (8 ounces, or 225 g) rinsed and drained shirataki rice (such as Miracle Rice), 1 cup (113 g) cauliflower rice, or 1 cup (186 g) cooked and cooled white or brown rice

Accessory needed:

Medium saucepan

Heat the olive oil in a medium saucepan over medium-high heat until it runs freely around the pan. Add the onion, garlic, salt, and turmeric. Sweat the onions until lightly translucent and fragrant, about 2 minutes.

Add the broth and chicken. Simmer for 10 minutes. Add the zucchini and shirataki rice and simmer for 4 minutes. Swirl 1 to 2 tablespoons (16 to 32 g) of pistou into each serving of the soup. Delish!

Nutritional Information: Calories: 194 – Protein: 22 g – Fat: 9.4 g – Carbs: 5.4 g – Fiber: 1.2 g – Net carbs: 4.2 g – Sodium: 904 mg – Potassium: 317 mg

1 cup (65 g) packed flat leaf parsley

1 clove garlic, minced

Zest of 1 lemon

⅔ cup (160 ml) extra virgin or light olive oil

½ teaspoon salt

Accessory needed:

Blender or food processor

Parsley Pistou

Total time: 3 minutes
Yield: 12 servings (2 tablespoons [24 g] each)

Combine all ingredients in a blender or food processor and blend until smooth.

Swirl a spoonful or two of pistou into each serving of soup and enjoy!

Red Lentil, Vegetable, and Coconut Soup

Originally, this was a clean-the-refrigerator soup from my days as a chef on private yachts, but it was such a hit that it became a regular in the meal rotation for both crew and guests! Loaded with micronutrients and anti-inflammatory ingredients, you can't go wrong with this filling, spicy, creamy soup.

Total time: 45 minutes   **Yield:** 6 servings

2 tablespoons (30 ml) coconut or extra-virgin olive oil

½ cup (80 g) chopped onion

1 tablespoon (10 g) minced garlic

2 tablespoons (12 g) minced ginger

Salt

½ cup (60 g) finely diced zucchini

½ cup (75 g) finely diced red pepper

½ cup (41 g) finely diced eggplant

½ cup (35 g) finely diced mushrooms

½ cup (65 g) finely chopped carrot

½ cup (50 g) finely chopped celery

1 cup (192 g) red lentils

4 cups (940 ml) vegetable or chicken bone broth

1 can (14.5 ounces, or 411 g) full-fat coconut milk

Black pepper

Accessory needed:

Large saucepan

Heat the oil in the saucepan over medium-high heat until it runs freely around the pan. Add the onion, garlic, ginger, and a pinch of salt and cook, stirring frequently, for about 5 minutes, until the onions start to become translucent.

Add the rest of the vegetables and cook until softened slightly, about 10 minutes. Stir in the lentils and combine well, cooking for 2 minutes. Pour in the broth and bring to a boil, stirring frequently to make sure the vegetables don't burn to the bottom of the pan. Lower the heat to medium and simmer for 15 minutes, continuing to stir regularly.

Once the lentils are soft, add the coconut milk and simmer for 5 to 10 minutes. Remove from the heat, season to taste, and enjoy!

Nutritional Information (using sugar): Calories: 340 – Protein: 16 g – Fat: 20 g – Carbs: 27 g – Fiber: 4.8 g – Net carbs: 22.2 g – Sodium: 352 mg – Potassium: 556 mg

Easy Antioxidant Pumpkin Tagine

I am keen on tagine! Moroccan spices bring out the best flavor in beta-carotene-rich pumpkin (or my favorite substitute, butternut squash). Combined with chickpeas and purple kale, you get a super dose of fiber and antioxidants in one vegetarian dish—and it really doesn't take that long to make.

Total time: 55 minutes   **Yield:** 4 servings

2 tablespoons (30 ml) extra-virgin olive oil

1 cup (128 g) large-dice onion

2 cloves garlic, peeled and sliced

1 tablespoon (6 g) minced ginger

Pinch of salt

3-4 cups (420–560 g) large-dice pumpkin or butternut squash

1 tablespoon (7 g) ras el hanout spice blend

3 cups (705 ml) vegetable broth, chicken broth, or water

1 can (14.5 ounces, or 411 g) diced tomatoes

1 can (14.5 ounces, or 411 g) chickpeas, drained and rinsed

1 tablespoon (15 ml) coconut aminos

1 bunch purple kale (green is fine if you can't find purple), torn into bite-size pieces

Rice or cauliflower rice

Accessory needed:

Large Dutch oven or lidded saucepan

Over medium-high heat, warm the olive oil in the pan until it flows easily. Add the onion, garlic, ginger, and a pinch of salt. Stir frequently for 5 minutes, making sure they don't burn. Stir in the pumpkin and ras el hanout. Cook for 5 minutes, then add the broth and tomatoes. Bring to a boil while stirring often, about 8 to 10 minutes. Lower the heat to medium, cover the pan, and cook for 10 minutes.

Remove the lid, stir to loosen anything starting to stick to the bottom of the pan, and check the doneness of the pumpkin. If it is easily pierced with a fork, add the chickpeas, coconut aminos, and kale. Simmer uncovered on the stovetop for 10 minutes. Remove from the heat and enjoy with a side of rice, another whole grain, or cauliflower rice.

Nutritional Information: Calories: 219 - Protein: 7.7 g - Fat: 9.3 g - Carbs: 30 g - Fiber: 8 g - Net carbs: 22 g - Sodium: 680 mg - Potassium: 788 mg

Green Turkey Chili & Limey Avocado-Onion Salad

Chili has always been a comfort food to me. This recipe fits that bill yet again, but with an incredible anti-inflammatory twist. Adding turmeric, two kinds of peppers, bone broth, and avocado take this from mere soup to superfood. You can add more traditional toppings such as sour cream, shredded cheese, or tortilla chips if you wish, but this lean turkey chili is scrumptious as is!

Total time: 40 minutes   **Yield:** 6 servings

½ cup (72 g) fresh poblano peppers (use canned, if necessary)

2 teaspoons (10 ml) avocado or extra-virgin olive oil

1 yellow onion, chopped (about 1 cup)

1 can (4 ounces, or 115 g) Hatch chiles (optional, but super yummy!)

Salt

1 pound (455 g) ground turkey

1 teaspoon ground cumin

1 teaspoon ground coriander

1 teaspoon turmeric

1 jar (16 ounces, or 455 g) mild green tomatillo salsa, also known as Mexican salsa verde

3 cups (705 ml) chicken bone broth

1 can (14 ounces, or 397 g) cannellini beans, drained and rinsed, and/or 2 cups (200 g) cauliflower florets, broken into small, bean-size pieces if keto/low carb

Black pepper

Sour cream and shredded cheese (optional)

Accessories needed:

Metal tongs

Large saucepan

Preheat the oven to 500°F (260°C, or gas mark 10).

Char the peppers on the stovetop over an open high flame, no pan necessary, using tongs to turn them as each side gets blackened and blistered but not ashen. This process takes only about 2 to 3 minutes per side. Transfer the blackened peppers to a resealable plastic bag or paper bag and seal tightly for 10 minutes to allow internal steam to help make the skin even more peel-able as well as cool them enough to handle. Once the peppers are cool enough to peel, slide the skins off. Remove the stem and seeds and chop into smallish dice, about ½-inch (1-cm) square.

In a large saucepan, heat the oil over medium-high heat until it shimmers and runs easily around the pan. Add the poblanos, onion, Hatch chiles (if using), and a pinch of salt. Sauté until the onions begin to turn translucent, about 4 minutes. Add the turkey and spices and combine well. Cook until the turkey is done, about 8 minutes, breaking the turkey into small pieces with a wooden spoon or spatula.

Pour in the salsa verde and bone broth and bring to a boil. Reduce the heat to medium and add the beans, cauliflower florets, or both depending on your preference! Simmer for 10 minutes before removing from the heat. Season with salt and pepper, and garnish with Limey Avocado-Onion Salad or sour cream and shredded cheese (if using).

Nutritional Information: Calories: 328 – Protein: 24 g – Fat: 15 g – Carbs: 25 g – Fiber: 6 g – Net carbs: 19 g – Sodium: 966 mg – Potassium: 822 mg

2 medium ripe avocadoes, chopped

1 small shallot, thinly sliced

2 tablespoons (2 g) cilantro leaves, roughly chopped

Juice of 1 lime

Salt and black pepper, to taste

Accessory needed:

Small mixing bowl

Limey Avocado-Onion Salad

Total time: 5 minutes
Yield: 6 servings

Chop avocadoes into ½-inch (1 cm) square pieces and place in a small mixing bowl. Add shallot, cilantro, and lime juice and combine well, keeping avocado mostly intact. Season with salt and black pepper to taste. Use as a topping for turkey chili, Bright Coriander Roasted Salmon (page 160), or really anything you like!

Easy Anti-Inflammatory Green Curry Soup

Did you know that curry paste is composed almost entirely of nutritional powerhouse ingredients? I especially love green curry with all its antioxidant fresh herbs, bloat- and anxiety-relieving lemongrass, anti-inflammatory roots such as galangal, turmeric, and ginger, and capsaicin-laced green peppers. Combined with MCT-containing coconut milk, bone broth, and green vegetables, every delicious spoonful brings you to next-level health while warming you up!

Total time: 40 minutes   **Yield:** 4 servings

¼ cup (64 g) Easy Mild Green Curry Paste (see note)

1 can (13.5 ounces, or 400 ml) full-fat coconut milk

2 teaspoons (6 g) coconut sugar, erythritol, or granulated monk fruit sweetener

1 teaspoon coconut aminos, tamari, or fish sauce

2 cups (475 ml) chicken bone broth or vegetable broth

½ cup (58 g) sliced onions

1 cup (90 g) chopped green cabbage or sliced Brussels sprouts

½ cup (50 g) chopped green beans, cut into 1-inch (2.5-cm) pieces

1 cup (71 g) fresh, bite-size broccoli florets

1 cup (70 g) sliced button mushrooms

Salt and black pepper

½ cup (8 g) fresh cilantro leaves

½ cup (24 g) fresh Thai basil

Accessory needed:

Large saucepan

In a large saucepan over medium-high heat, whisk together the curry paste, coconut milk, sweetener, coconut aminos, and broth. Bring the mixture to a light boil and then reduce the heat to low. Allow the mixture to reduce for 5 minutes, stirring occasionally.

Add the onions and cabbage. Cover and simmer for 10 minutes, until the onions are soft and the cabbage is becoming tender. Add the green beans, broccoli, and mushrooms, then cover and cook for 5 minutes. The beans and broccoli should be bright green and crisp-tender. The mushrooms will just be getting soft.

Season with salt and pepper to taste. Divide among four serving bowls, and garnish with basil and cilantro leaves.

Nutritional Information: Calories: 275 – Protein: 9.2 g – Fat: 22 g – Carbs: 15 g – Fiber: 2.5 g – Net carbs: 6.5 g (due to sugar alcohol adjustment) – Sodium: 798 mg – Potassium: 529 mg

Note:

You can use prepared Thai green curry paste purchased at the grocery store or online, but there is nothing more delicious than freshly made.

Dairy-Free Creamy Cauliflower Soup

Cauliflower is one of my favorite vegetables for a zillion healthy reasons: It's known to protect against cancer, has mood-boosting B-vitamins, and is a great source of fiber to name a few of them! This soup is simple and creamy without any added dairy or coconut cream. The creaminess comes from the good fats! Because we blend in extra MCT oil at the end, it's a quick energy booster, too.

Total time: 30 minutes   **Yield:** 4 servings

2 tablespoons (30 ml) extra-virgin olive oil

1 cup (160 g) finely chopped onion

1 bay leaf

Salt

1–2 pounds (455–910 g) cauliflower florets and stems

4 cups (940 ml) chicken bone broth or water

1 tablespoon (15 ml) MCT oil

Black pepper

Lemon juice and crushed red pepper flakes (optional)

Accessories needed:

Saucepan

Blender or immersion blender

In a saucepan over medium-high heat, warm the olive oil until it runs freely around the pan. Add the onion, bay leaf, and a pinch of salt, sweating the onion for 5 minutes until it starts to become soft and translucent.

Add the cauliflower and broth and bring to a boil for 5 minutes. Reduce the heat to medium and cook until the cauliflower is soft, about 10 minutes. Add the MCT oil and blend. Season with salt and pepper to taste and divide among 4 serving bowls. Garnish with a spritz of lemon juice and a sprinkle of crushed red pepper flakes (if using).

Nutritional Information (with 2 pounds [910 g] cauliflower & chicken bone broth): Calories: 188 – Protein: 17 g – Fat: 11 g – Carbs: 14 g – Fiber: 6 g – Net carbs: 8 g – Sodium: 361 mg – Potassium: 982 mg

Chilled Avocado Soup

This is unlike any chilled avocado soup you have had—it tastes more like a salad! It's nutritious and nourishing, and your skin will glow like nothing before. Avocado, spinach, grapefruit, and walnuts are all known to supply radiant skin, and the collagen in bone broth is great for not just your skin, but hair and nails, as well.

Total time: 40 minutes (including chilling time) **Yield:** 4 servings

3 cups (705 ml) chicken bone broth or vegetable broth

2 ripe medium Hass avocados, peeled and pitted

2 cups (60 g) baby spinach

¼ cup (60 ml) fresh pink grapefruit juice (from about ½ a grapefruit)

2 green onions, chopped

1 tablespoon (15 ml) white wine or champagne vinegar

1 tablespoon (15 ml) extra-virgin olive oil

Salt and black pepper

Toasted walnuts and crumbled feta (optional)

Accessory needed:

Blender

Combine the broth, avocados, spinach, grapefruit juice, green onions, vinegar, and oil in a blender. Puree until smooth. Season with the salt and pepper to taste. Chill until you are ready to serve.

Divide among four serving bowls and garnish with toasted walnuts and feta crumbles, if desired.

Nutritional Information (without garnish): Calories: 187 – Protein: 9 g – Fat: 14 g – Carbs: 8.8 g – Fiber: 5.1 g – Net carbs: 3.7 g – Sodium: 383 mg – Potassium: 492 mg

Salads

SALADS FOREVER! Salads are not just for hot days, especially when they're as hearty, colorful, and balanced as these are. Salads in general are amazing sources of fiber, nutrients, and hydration through food—keeping our digestion going and skin glowing! By adding high-quality protein and healthy fat, we have the opportunity to give our body a complete, delicious meal.

Raid the pantry and take care of the hangries quickly with Tuna Chickpea Parsley Salad (page 99). Make your coworkers totally jealous while using up the last of your rotisserie chicken with a Fast & Filling Low-Carb Vietnamese Chicken and Cabbage Salad (page 109), one of my personal go-to meals. Or get a little tropical with Satay Shrimp & Crunchy Rainbow Slaw (page 104)! You'll be a salad convert in no time.

Tuna Chickpea Parsley Salad

This salad comes together so fast, you will forget how little time it took to make by the time you finish it! Pair it with a few lettuce leaves or a pita pocket to make it extra lunchy. Tuna is an abundant source of protein, omega-3 fatty acids, selenium, and vitamin D. Chickpeas provide fiber, potassium, B vitamins, iron, and magnesium. Parsley is a vitamin K–rich leafy green. Together in one bowl, you almost couldn't ask for something more nutritious!

Total time: 10 minutes **Yield:** 2 servings

1 can (5 ounces, or 140 g) solid white albacore tuna, drained

1 can (14 ounces, or 397 g) chickpeas, drained and rinsed

¼ cup (40 g) finely diced red onion

1 bunch fresh parsley, leaves only

2 tablespoons (30 ml) extra-virgin olive oil

1 tablespoon (15 ml) balsamic vinegar

Salt and black pepper

Accessory needed:

Medium mixing bowl

Place the tuna, chickpeas, and onion in the bowl and mash together with a fork. It can be chunky—leave larger pieces of tuna and plenty of chickpeas unmashed. Stir in the parsley, olive oil, and balsamic vinegar. Season to taste with salt and pepper.

Nutritional Information: Calories: 423 - Protein: 23 g – Fat: 19 g – Carbs: 42 g – Fiber: 11 g – Net carbs: 31 g – Sodium: 768 mg – Potassium: 563 mg

Baby Spinach, Blueberry, and Goat Cheese Salad with Crispy Tempeh

Baby spinach, blueberries, and goat cheese are heavenly on their own, but the addition of slightly crispy, savory tempeh crumbles makes this a full protein-laden vegetarian meal.

Total time: 35 minutes   **Yield:** 2 servings

Crispy Tempeh

2 cups (475 ml) water

½ teaspoon salt

1 block (8 ounces, or 225 g) tempeh

2 teaspoons (10 ml) avocado or extra-virgin olive oil

¼ teaspoon dried thyme

¼ teaspoon paprika

Salt and black pepper

1 tablespoon (15 ml) coconut aminos or tamari

Dressing

2 tablespoons (30 ml) raspberry vinegar

2 tablespoons (30 ml) olive oil

¼ teaspoon Dijon mustard

Pinch each salt and pepper

Salad

4 cups (120 g) baby spinach

¼ cup (38 g) crumbled goat cheese

¼ cup (38 g) blueberries

¼ cup (30 g) toasted walnut halves

2 tablespoons (20 g) sliced shallot

Accessories needed:

Small frying pan

Small jar with a tight-fitting lid

Make the crispy tempeh: Add the water and salt to the frying pan over high heat. Bring to a boil and reduce the heat to medium. Add the tempeh and simmer for 10 minutes before draining and setting on a plate to cool. Wash out the pan. Crumble the tempeh into pieces, preferably ¼- to ½-inch (3- to 6-mm). The smaller the pieces, the crispier they will get.

Return the frying pan to the stove over medium-high heat and add the oil, heating it until it runs freely around the pan. Add the tempeh and spices and stir frequently for 5 to 7 minutes, until the tempeh is lightly browned all over. Stir in the coconut aminos and cook for 2 minutes or so, until there is no liquid left. Remove from the heat and set aside to cool slightly. Season with salt and pepper.

Make the dressing: In a small screw-top jar, combine all the dressing ingredients. Secure the lid and shake until emulsified.

Make the salad: Divide the fresh salad ingredients between two plates or containers. Sprinkle each with half of the tempeh crumbles and half the dressing.

Nutritional Information: Calories: 518 – Protein: 30.5 g – Fat: 37 g – Carbs: 27 g – Fiber: 15 g – Net carbs: 12 g – Sodium: 320 mg – Potassium: 1417 mg

Poached Chicken and Arugula Salad with Bistro Vinaigrette

This dish tastes like lunch in the South of France. With the delicate flavor of poached chicken offset by peppery arugula and a bold bistro vinaigrette, you might feel like you should be looking at a vineyard instead of sitting at home or work.

Total time: 23 minutes **Yield:** 2 servings

Salad

2 cups (475 ml) water

5 black peppercorns

½ teaspoon salt

1 bay leaf

1 (8 ounces, or 225 g) chicken breast

2 tablespoons (14 g) shaved almonds

4 cups (80 g) baby arugula

¼ cup (20 g) thinly sliced red shallot

2 tablespoons (15 g) roasted pepper strips (I like yellow for this salad)

Dressing

¼ teaspoon fine salt

1 small clove garlic, minced (about ½ teaspoon)

2 tablespoons (30 ml) white wine or champagne vinegar

3 tablespoons (45 ml) extra-virgin olive oil

¼ teaspoon Dijon mustard

Accessories needed:

Small saucepan or deep-sided small frying pan

Pie tin

Mortar and pestle or blender

Medium mixing bowl

Preheat the oven to 400°F (200°C, or gas mark 6).

Make the salad: Over high heat, bring the water, salt, peppercorns, and bay leaf to a boil. Reduce the heat to low and add the chicken. Simmer for 15 minutes and remove from the heat. Cool in cooking liquid for 10 minutes before draining. Slice into thin pieces.

Add the almonds to a pie tin, place in the oven, and toast for 5 minutes. Remove from the oven and set aside. Pro-tip: Set a timer! Even chefs overcook a lot of nuts!

Traditional dressing method: Combine salt and garlic in a mortar and mash into a paste with a pestle. Add the vinegar and scrape down the sides with a fork. Use the fork to whisk in the oil and Dijon mustard until it is emulsified.

Quick dressing method: Place all dressing ingredients into a blender and pulse until emulsified.

Transfer chicken to a medium mixing bowl. Add the arugula, shallot, and roasted pepper. Drizzle with dressing and season with salt and pepper. Divide the salad among two serving plates and garnish with toasted almonds.

Nutritional Information: Calories: 242 - Protein: 30 g - Fat: 8.2 g - Carbs: 14 g - Fiber: 5.3 g - Net carbs: 8.7 g - Sodium: 648 mg - Potassium: 814 mg

Satay Shrimp & Crunchy Rainbow Slaw

Satay where you are! Because you're gonna love this one. Satay sauce usually involves peanut butter, and that is totally a possibility, but this dressing works just as well with almond or sunflower seed butters. Probably even better, though I haven't tried them yet!

Total time: 30 minutes   **Yield:** 2 servings

Shrimp

8 ounces (225 g) raw shrimp, peeled, no smaller than 26-30

2 teaspoons (10 ml) avocado oil or another neutral oil

2 teaspoons (10 ml) coconut aminos or tamari

2 teaspoons (4 g) minced fresh ginger

½ teaspoon ground turmeric

½ teaspoon ground coriander

¼ teaspoon fine salt

Dressing

¼ cup (65 g) creamy plain nut or seed butter (peanut, almond, cashew, sun butter)

¼ cup (60 ml) coconut milk

2 tablespoons (20 g) minced shallot or white part of green onion

1 tablespoon (9 g) coconut sugar, maple syrup, yacon syrup, or maple-flavored monk fruit syrup

1 tablespoon (15 ml) fresh lime juice

1 tablespoon (15 ml) soy sauce, tamari, or coconut aminos

1 tablespoon (15 ml) sambal or sriracha

1 teaspoon minced fresh ginger

Slaw

1 cup (70 g) shredded red cabbage

1 bunch curly kale, torn into bite-size pieces

1 medium carrot, julienned (about ½ cup)

½ small sweet red bell pepper, julienned (about ½ cup)

½ cup (70 g) chopped cucumber

¼ cup (35 g) chopped salted roasted almonds

1 green onion, sliced on the bias

Accessories needed:

Medium mixing bowl

Small skewers

Large mixing bowl

Blender

Cast-iron or nonstick frying pan

Make the shrimp: In a medium mixing bowl, combine all of the shrimp ingredients and toss well to coat evenly. Thread 2 to 4 shrimp on each skewer depending on size. Set aside to marinate on the skewers in the mixing bowl while you prepare the slaw.

Make the dressing: With clean hands, add all the dressing ingredients to a blender and blend at high speed until smooth. This will make about 1 cup, plus extra!

Make the slaw: In a large mixing bowl, combine all of the slaw ingredients and ¼ cup (60 ml) of the satay sauce. Toss well to incorporate. Set aside.

Heat the frying pan over medium-high heat until a drop of water sizzles upon contact, about 3 minutes. Place the skewers into the pan in a single layer. Do not crowd the pan or you will not get the crispy browned edges that we are going for. Cook for 2 to 3 minutes on each side, flipping only once. They should curl up and brown a little on each side. Remove from the pan to a plate as soon as they are done.

Divide the slaw between 2 plates and top with half of the skewers. Drizzle 1 tablespoon (15 ml) of dressing over the shrimp, and garnish with a sprinkle of green onions.

Nutritional Information (using maple syrup):
Calories: 370 – Protein: 23 g – Fat: 19.5 g – Carbs: 20 g – Fiber: 5.4 g – Net carbs: 14.6 g – Sodium: 112 mg – Potassium: 445 mg

Black Rice and Brussels Sprout Waldorf Salad

Black rice, also known as forbidden rice, is a nutritious powerhouse with tons of antioxidant plant pigments called anthocyanins and a nutty, chewy texture similar to brown rice. It brings this salad to a new level of complexity and heartiness, making it a truly filling meal!

Total time: 60 minutes   **Yield:** 4 servings

Rice

½ cup (90 g) black or wild rice

1 ½ cups (355 ml) cold water

Pinch of salt

Dressing

½ cup (115 g) full-fat plain yogurt or sour cream

¼ cup (60 ml) buttermilk

¼ cup (60 ml) apple cider vinegar

1 tablespoon (4 g) chopped fresh dill

Salt and black pepper

Salad

½ cup (60 g) walnut halves

8 ounces (225 g) Brussels sprouts, sliced thinly or shaved with a mandoline

1 cup (100 g) celery, sliced ¼-inch (6 mm) thick on the bias (diagonally)

½ cup (55 g) finely chopped or julienned apple

½ cup (55 g) finely chopped or julienned pear

2 green onions, chopped, both white and green parts

Accessories needed:

Small saucepan with lid

Small bowl

Pie tin

Large mixing bowl

Baking tray

Heat the oven to 400°F (200°C, or gas mark 6).

Make the rice: Combine the rice, water, and salt in a small saucepan over high heat and bring to a boil. Reduce the heat to low and simmer, covered, for 50 minutes.

Make the dressing: While the rice cooks, in a small bowl, combine all ingredients for the dressing and whisk together. Set aside.

Make the salad: Place walnut halves in a pie tin and toast for 5 minutes once the oven comes up to temperature. Make sure you set a timer! Remove from oven and cool completely.

Add the raw fruit and vegetables to a large mixing bowl. Once the rice is cooked, tip it onto a plate or baking tray and spread in a thin layer to speed cooling. As soon as it stops steaming, add it to the large mixing bowl along with the walnuts. Pour over the dressing and fold in gently. Serve at your leisure—though it will be hard to resist!

Nutritional Information: Calories: 187 – Protein: 6.8 g – Fat: 9.4 g – Carbs: 21 g – Fiber: 4.6 g – Net carbs: 16.4 g – Sodium: 90 mg – Potassium: 510 mg

Fast & Filling Low-Carb Vietnamese Chicken and Cabbage Salad

You won't be able to get enough of this crunchy, spicy, flavorful salad! It's low in carbs and high in fiber. If that isn't enough, it is so shortcut-friendly that you can have it in a bowl and on your table in about 10 minutes. You can shred a rotisserie chicken breast, use a prepared coleslaw mix, pre-shredded carrots, and salted roasted peanuts to cut prep time in half. Even if you don't, it *still* comes together quickly!

Total time: 10 minutes   **Yield:** 4 servings

Salad

2 cups (280 g) cooked, shredded chicken breast

3 cups (210 g) very finely shredded cabbage (I like a mix of red and green.)

1 cup (110 g) shredded carrot

1 cup (96 g) thinly sliced mint leaves

1 stalk lemongrass, very finely minced

½ cup (24 g) fresh Thai basil or laksa leaves, thinly sliced

¼ cup (36 g) chopped roasted peanuts

Dressing

3 tablespoons (45 ml) fish sauce

¼ cup (45 ml) lime or lemon juice

1 tablespoon (15 g) erythritol, granulated monk fruit, or sugar

1 tablespoon (10 g) minced garlic

2 Thai bird's eye chiles, crumbled or ¼ teaspoon crushed red pepper

Accessories needed:

Large and small mixing bowls

Make the salad: Combine all of the salad ingredients in a large mixing bowl. Toss well.

Make the dressing: Whisk together the dressing ingredients in a smaller bowl.

Pour over the salad ingredients. Toss well to combine and enjoy, just like that!

Nutritional Information (using sugar):
Calories: 213 – Protein: 23 g – Fat: 9 g – Carbs: 12 g – Fiber: 4 g – Net carbs: 8.8 g – Sodium: 310 mg – Potassium: 553 mg

Thai Beef Salad with Fresh Herbs & Umami-Lime Dressing

Did you know that fresh herbs count as dark leafy greens? Cilantro in particular is one of the greatest detoxifiers we can consume. This flavor-packed salad is as good for you as it gets, sky-high in satiating protein and fiber with a little kick of heat that will get your motor running.

Total time: 20 minutes   **Yield:** 4 servings

1 pound (455 g) flank steak

1 tablespoon (15 ml) coconut aminos, tamari, or soy sauce

1 teaspoon avocado oil

Zest of 1 lime

Juice of 1 lime (about 2-3 tablespoons [30-45 ml])

2 tablespoons (30 ml) fish sauce

1 teaspoon coconut sugar, palm sugar, granulated monk fruit or erythritol

1 stem lemongrass, white part only, chopped very fine

1 Thai bird's eye chile, sliced thinly

2-3 tablespoons (20-30 g) thinly sliced shallot

2 green onions, thinly sliced on the bias

½ cup (48 g) fresh mint leaves, roughly chopped

½ cup (8 g) fresh cilantro leaves, roughly chopped

½ cup (24 g) fresh Thai basil or regular basil, roughly chopped (optional)

½ cup (62 g) quartered grape or cherry tomatoes

½ cup (70 g) deseeded sliced cucumber

2 cups (140 g) shredded green cabbage

1 packet (7 ounces, or 196 g) rinsed and drained shirataki angel hair (such as Miracle Noodle)

Salt and black pepper

Accessories needed:

Edged plate or resealable plastic bag for marinating

Nonstick frying pan

Medium mixing bowl

Alternative Method

More traditionally, all of the ingredients of this salad—vegetables, beef, juices from sliced beef, and lime dressing—are combined in one bowl at the same time and served. You, too, can do this and it will taste absolutely divine! I break it down into the steps I have to make it more transportable and extra pleasing to the eye.

Thai Beef Salad with Fresh Herbs & Umami-Lime Dressing (continued from page 110)

Marinate the steak in a mixture of coconut aminos, avocado oil, and lime zest for 10 minutes minimum.

While that is marinating, whisk together the lime juice, fish sauce, and sugar in a small mixing bowl until the sugar is dissolved. Set aside.

Place in a nonstick frying pan over medium heat and stir until the noodles are dry and turn pretty opaque white, about 5 minutes. Transfer to medium mixing bowl and allow to cool while you wash the frying pan and replace on the stove over medium-high heat.

By the time the pan comes up to temperature (when a drop of water sizzles upon contact), the steak will have been marinating for 10 minutes. Place it in the pan and cook on each side for 4 to 5 minutes per side for medium-rare beef. Once both sides are cooked and lightly browned, remove from the pan and set aside on a plate. Cover with foil to rest for 10 minutes.

As the meat rests, add all the raw vegetables and herbs to the mixing bowl with the noodles. Combine evenly and divide among four plates.

Slice the meat as thinly as you can against the grain and top each plate (or meal prep container!) with one-quarter of the steak. Pour approximately 1 tablespoon (15 ml) of dressing over each serving to be consumed immediately.

Nutritional Information: Calories: 268 – Protein: 25 g – Fat: 10 g – Carbs: 6.25 g – Fiber: 2.5 g – Net carbs: 3.75 g – Sodium: 482 mg – Potassium: 106 mg

Warm Quinoa, Chard, and Chickpea Salad

Greens and beans and quinoa! This is a hearty, nutritious vegan bowl packed with plant protein and fiber. It can be eaten warm or cold, and it even slides nicely into a warm bowl of broth should you feel so inclined.

Total time: 30 minutes   **Yield:** 4 servings

1 cup (173 g) dry quinoa

2 cups (475 ml) vegetable stock or water

Salt or a splash of coconut aminos

2 tablespoons (30 ml) extra-virgin olive oil

1 red onion, chopped small

1 bunch Swiss chard (silver beet) chopped, stems and leaves separated

¼ teaspoon garlic powder or granulated garlic

Zest and juice of 1 lemon

1 can (15 ounces, or 425 g) chickpeas, drained and rinsed

Salt and black pepper

Accessories needed:

Fine-mesh sieve

Small saucepan with lid or rice cooker

Large frying pan

Rinse the quinoa in the fine-mesh sieve until the water runs clear. This will produce a fluffier quinoa. Transfer the quinoa, stock, and a pinch of salt to the small saucepan. Bring to a boil over medium-high heat before reducing temperature to medium-low and simmering until all the liquid is absorbed, about 15 to 20 minutes. Remove from the heat when this is done.

While that cooks, warm the olive oil in the frying pan over medium-high heat until it flows easily around the pan. Add the onion, Swiss chard stems, garlic powder, and a pinch of salt. Sauté, stirring frequently, until the onion begins to become translucent and the chard stems have softened slightly, about 4 minutes. Reduce the heat to medium-low and stir in the chard leaves to wilt, adding the lemon juice to steam through.

Add the chickpeas and turn heat to low until the quinoa is finished cooking. Add the quinoa and lemon zest to the green-and-bean mixture, and season with salt and pepper.

Nutritional Information: Calories: 410 – Protein: 17 g – Fat: 12 g – Carbs: 61 g – Fiber: 12 g – Net carbs: 49 g – Sodium: 621 mg – Potassium: 900 mg

Superfood Salmon Niçoise with Black Lentils

I've taken the standard Niçoise up a notch by swapping in superfood salmon for tuna, purple potatoes for regular, and adding extra nutritious black lentils! You still get that classic South of France feeling, but with a healthy happy twist. Salmon and lentils are both known for their mood-boosting properties, so why *not* get happy while eating this protein-packed dish?

Total time: 55 minutes   **Yield:** 2 servings

Salad

½ cup (96 g) black lentils

Salt

Black pepper

4 ounces (115 g) purple potatoes, sliced into ½-inch (1-cm) rounds

4 ounces (115 g) fresh green beans, broken into bite-size pieces

8 ounces (225 g) salmon fillet

¼ teaspoon herbs de Provence

2 cups (110 g) romaine lettuce torn into bite-size pieces

2 cups (275 ml) water

1 hard-boiled egg, chopped

½ cup (62 g) chopped cherry tomatoes

1½ (355 ml) cups water

¼ teaspoon salt

2 tablespoons (40 g) prepared olive tapenade (such as Divina)

Lemon wedges

Dressing

2 tablespoons (30 ml) extra-virgin olive oil

2 tablespoons (30 ml) white wine vinegar

½ teaspoon Dijon mustard, preferably grainy

½ teaspoon minced garlic

Accessories needed:

Small saucepan

Medium saucepan

Strainer

Parchment paper

Pie tin or baking tray

2-quart (2 L) saucepan

Large mixing bowl

Preheat the oven to 425°F (220°C, or gas mark 6).

Make the salad: Sift through lentils and rinse until the water runs clear. Place into a small saucepan with 1½ cups (355 ml) of water and a pinch of salt and bring to a boil. Reduce the heat to low and simmer, covered, for 22 minutes. Remove cover and let cool slightly.

Meanwhile, place the potatoes and 2 cups (475 ml) of water into a medium saucepan with a pinch of salt and bring to a boil over medium-high heat. Reduce the heat to medium-low and simmer until the potatoes are just easily pierced with a fork, about 10 minutes. Add the green beans to the potato pan and simmer for 1 to 2 minutes, when the beans are bright green and crisp-tender. Transfer to a strainer in the sink to drain and cool.

Place the salmon on a parchment-lined pie tin and drizzle with ½ teaspoon olive oil. Season with herbs de Provence, salt and pepper to taste. Bake for 12 minutes. Remove and set aside.

Make the dressing: Whisk together the dressing ingredients in a small bowl or shake in a small screw-top jar to emulsify.

In a large mixing bowl, combine the romaine, tomatoes, egg, potatoes, green beans, lentils, tapenade, and dressing. Season with salt and pepper. Divide mixture between 2 plates and top each with half of the salmon. Garnish with lemon wedges.

Nutritional Information: Calories: 545 – Protein: 42 g – Fat: 25 g – Carbs: 39 g – Fiber: 11 g – Net carbs: 28 g – Sodium: 775 mg – Potassium: 1640 mg

Miso-Glazed Tofu and Gingery Green Bean Salad

Talk about a high-protein vegetarian meal with lots of flavor! The marinade doubles as a dressing with healthy, fermented miso paste. There are a few steps to this dish, but they're all easy and worth it when you take your first bite. No more sad desk lunches here!

Total time: 45 minutes   **Yield:** 2 servings

Marinade/Dressing

¼ cup (64 g) miso paste

¼ cup (60 ml) coconut aminos

¼ cup (60 ml) rice wine vinegar

3 tablespoons (45 ml) avocado oil

2 teaspoons (6 g) minced garlic

2 teaspoons (4 g) minced ginger

⅔ cup (110 g) chopped onion

Tofu

1 block (10 ounces, or 280 g)
extra-firm tofu (such as Hodo)

½ recipe marinade

Gingery Green Beans

8 ounces (225 g) fresh green beans,
broken into bite-size pieces

2 cups (475 ml) water

Pinch salt

1 tablespoon (6 g) minced ginger

1 tablespoon (15 ml) avocado oil

Salt and black pepper

Accessories needed:

Blender

Baking tray

Parchment paper

Small mixing bowl

Medium saucepan

Strainer

Small frying pan

Preheat the oven to 400°F (200°C, or gas mark 6). Line a baking tray with parchment paper.

Make the dressing: Combine all the dressing ingredients in a blender and process until smooth.

Make the tofu: Cut the block of tofu into ½- x 1-inch (1- x 2.5-cm) pieces. Add it to the baking tray and toss with half of the dressing mixture. Bake for 20 minutes, flipping once halfway. Remove and allow to cool for 5 minutes.

Make the green beans: While the tofu bakes, bring 2 cups (475 ml) of water to a boil with a pinch of salt. Blanch the beans for 1 to 2 minutes, until bright green and crisp tender. Strain and transfer to a small mixing bowl.

Warm the tablespoon of oil in a small frying pan over medium heat until it flows around the pan freely. Add the minced ginger and sauté until fragrant but not browning, about 2 minutes. Remove from the heat and cool slightly. Pour over the cooked green beans, and season with salt and pepper.

Divide the green beans between two plates and top each with half of the tofu. Drizzle 1 tablespoon of marinade/dressing over each dish. Enjoy warm or cold.

Nutritional Information: Calories: 441 – Protein: 27 g – Fat: 27 g – Carbs: 24 g – Fiber: 9 g – Net carbs: 15 g – Sodium: 600 mg – Potassium: 48 mg

Lunches

Lunch is oftentimes the "breakfast" of the world of intermittent fasting, so we want to make sure that it is absolutely crush-worthy! No sad desk lunches here—more like #brunchlife every day. The key to lunch perfection is a rainbow of colors and a broad range of textures to satisfy all the senses AND your body's needs, especially in a more public setting because we're often eating among friends and coworkers.

Feel like you're splurging—and be sure to plan ahead for the office pizza party—with Barbecue Chicken and Charred Onion Personal Pizzas (page 119). Keep it light-but-luxe with an Asparagus and Goat Cheese Frittata with Fresh Herb Salad (page 129), also perfect for entertaining! Every option will leave you loving lunch more.

Barbecue Chicken and Charred Onion Personal Pizzas

Who doesn't love pizza? This one has a crust made out of cheese and almonds, and the taste and crispy texture are so satisfying that you may want to have it every day of the week. As one recipe is enough for six servings, you could absolutely do that! Or just freeze the dough for a later date and try out new topping combinations on a whim.

Total time: 40 minutes   **Yield:** 6 servings

Almond Mozzarella Crust

2 cups (230 g) shredded mozzarella

1½ cups (156 g) almond flour

¼ cup (60 g) cream cheese, cut into small cubes

1½ tablespoons (21 g) baking powder

1 egg

Pizzas

1½ cups (270 g) shredded chicken
(poached or from a rotisserie chicken)

¼ cup (40 g) red onion

½ tablespoon (8 ml) extra-virgin olive oil

¼ teaspoon fine salt

1½ cups (175 g) shredded Monterey Jack
or Mozzarella cheese

2 tablespoons (30 ml) prepared barbecue sauce of
your choosing (I use G. Hughes Sugar Free.)

Accessories needed:

Large microwave-safe mixing bowl

Microwave

Parchment paper

Rolling pin

2 baking trays

Frying pan

Barbecue Chicken and Charred Onion Personal Pizzas (continued from page 119)

Preheat the oven to 400°F (200°C, or gas mark 6).

Make the crust: In a microwave safe bowl, combine the mozzarella, almond flour, cream cheese, and baking powder. Combine well by stirring with a fork and then cook in the microwave at high power for 1 minute. Remove, and stir again with a fork, repeating the process with 30-second intervals afterward until all the cheese shreds are indistinguishable and a large ball of dough is formed. Allow to cool for a few minutes so that you can easily handle the dough. Crack an egg into the cheese and almond mixture and knead until the egg is fully combined. Place the bowl into the refrigerator to cool for 10 minutes.

Make the pizza: While the dough chills, heat the oil in a small frying pan over medium-high heat until the oil runs easily around the pan. Add the onions and ¼ teaspoon salt and sauté, stirring frequently, until the onions begin to become translucent. Lower the heat to medium-low and allow to cook, stirring occasionally, until they start to brown about 5 minutes. Remove pan from heat and set aside.

Take dough out of fridge and split into 6 equal portions, rolling each one into a smooth ball before replacing in the bowl for organization's sake. Line 2 baking trays with parchment paper and set aside. Then, on a flat surface, lay out one extra-long (about 24 inches or 60 cm) piece of parchment paper that can fold over itself to form a 12-inch (30-cm) packet. Place a dough ball in the middle of the top half and fold paper upward to cover, pressing down on the ball to flatten into a disc.

Use a rolling pin to roll this out to about a ½-inch (1-cm) thickness, making a 6- to 8-inch (15- to 20-cm) pizza base. Transfer to the waiting baking tray and repeat the process with the rest of the dough. You should be able to fit 3 bases per standard baking tray.

Spread 1 teaspoon of the prepared barbecue sauce on each one. Top with one-sixth of the cheese, chicken, and cooked onions. Bake for 15 to 18 minutes, until the bottom of the crust is golden, and the cheese is starting to brown on top.

Nutritional Information: Calories: 438 – Protein: 28 g – Fat: 31 g – Carbs: 15 g – Fiber: 3.7 g – Net carbs: 11.3 g – Sodium: 921 mg – Potassium: 394 mg

Note:

Note: these can be made, cooled, frozen, and reheated for 15 minutes at 350° (180°C, or gas mark 4) if you so desire. They're great to have on hand to pop into a toaster oven when you're short on time!

Turkey-Provolone-Roasted Red Pepper Lettuce Wraps with Quick Basil Aioli

This is one of my go-to meals and ideal for quick meal prep. It comes together in a heartbeat and is portable and low-carb to boot, keeping those pesky sugar cravings at bay. The quick basil aioli will undoubtedly become an instant favorite you will want to smother on *everything*.

Total time: 10 minutes   **Yield:** 4 servings (2 wraps per serving)

Quick Basil Aioli

½ cup (115 g) prepared mayonnaise

1 clove garlic

2 tablespoons (30 ml) fresh lemon juice (about ½ a lemon)

¼ cup (12 g) loosely packed fresh basil

Lettuce Wraps

8 butter, green, or red lettuce leaves

8 slices (1 ounce, or 28 g each) slices provolone

16 slices (1 ounce, or 28 g each) roasted turkey breast

8 teaspoons Quick Basil Aioli

½ cup (90 g) roasted red pepper strips

Accessory needed:

Blender

Make the Quick Basil Aioli: Combine all ingredients in a blender and blend until smooth.

Make the Lettuce Wraps: If you have a large enough workspace, this recipe is best done all at the same time to make things easier. Lay out the lettuce leaves individually. Top each leaf with a slice of provolone, followed by two slices of turkey, 1 teaspoon of aioli, and one-quarter of the pepper strips.

Roll into cylinders and enjoy! To store/pack/plate, place with the seam-side down so they don't unroll. Keep a little of that extra aioli on hand for dipping, too!

Nutritional Information: Calories: 341 – Protein: 42 g – Fat: 17 g – Carbs: 2.9 g – Fiber: 0.4 g – Net carbs: 2.5 g – Sodium: 627 mg – Potassium: 426 mg

Protein-Packed Thai Pork in Lettuce Bowls

This filling, nutritious minced pork salad features all of the traditional Thai flavorings (each with its own health benefits!) and a vitamin C–laden lime dressing. It comes together quickly and on a budget. Here, we use ground pork, but feel free to try this one with chicken, turkey, or beef.

Total time: 30 minutes   **Yield:** 4 servings

1 tablespoon (15 ml) avocado oil

1 pound (455 g) ground pork

1 stalk finely chopped lemongrass, white part only

1 tablespoon (6 g) minced ginger

2 small cloves garlic, crushed

Salt

1 can water chestnuts (optional, but adds a nice crunchy texture), drained and chopped into small dice

½ cup (48 g) chopped fresh mint

¼ cup (4 g) chopped fresh cilantro leaves

Black pepper

2 tablespoons (30 ml) fish sauce, tamari, or coconut aminos

3 tablespoons (45 ml) fresh squeezed lime juice

3 green onions, sliced thinly on the diagonal

2 shallots, sliced thin

12 full butter lettuce leaves

1 carrot, julienned

1 cucumber, peeled, seeded, and chopped into small dice

2 tablespoons (18 g) chopped roasted, salted almonds

Accessories needed:

Frying pan

Medium mixing bowl

In a frying pan, heat the avocado oil over medium-high heat until it flows freely around the pan. Lower the heat to medium and add the pork, lemongrass, ginger, garlic, and a pinch of salt. Break apart the meat with a wooden spoon or spatula and make sure the fragrant additions get well incorporated. Stir frequently until the pork is cooked through, about 10 minutes. Remove from the heat and set aside to cool for 5 minutes.

In a medium mixing bowl, add the water chestnuts (if using), mint, and cilantro. Add the pork mixture, fish sauce, and lime juice. Combine thoroughly and adjust the seasoning with salt and pepper.

Place about one-quarter of the mixture in each lettuce leaf. Arrange julienned carrot, sliced shallot, and diced cucumber on top and enjoy taco style!

Nutritional Information: Calories: 420 – Protein: 23 g – Fat: 30 g – Carbs: 16 g – Fiber: 4 g – Net carbs: 12 g – Sodium: 829 mg – Potassium: 826 mg

Crispy Turnip Hash Browns & Cumin Roasted Vegetables in a Southwestern Yogurt Sauce

This is one rainbow-colored flavor combination that you don't want to miss. The roasted vegetables come together with the cumin well, and they are complemented by the contrasting textures and flavors of the slightly crispy hash browns and cool, spiced yogurt sauce.

Total time: 50 minutes   **Yield:** 4 servings

Cumin-Roasted Vegetables

1 cup (71 g) broccoli florets, broken into small pieces

1 cup (150 g) chopped sweet bell pepper

1 cup chopped yellow squash or zucchini (about 8 ounces, or 225 g)

½ cup (80 g) chopped onion

1 tablespoon (15 ml) extra-virgin olive oil

1 teaspoon ground cumin

½ teaspoon cumin seeds (optional but awesome!)

¼ teaspoon salt

Freshly ground black pepper

Turnip Hash Browns

1 egg

⅛ teaspoon salt

⅛ teaspoon pepper

1 pound (455 g) turnips (about 2–3 medium to large ones)

2 tablespoons (28 g) butter, ghee, bacon fat, or tallow, divided

Southwestern Yogurt Sauce

1 container (5 ounces, or 140 g) or heaping ½ cup plain yogurt of your choice

¼ teaspoon prepared chili powder

Salt

Accessories needed:

Baking tray

Parchment paper

2 large mixing bowls

Frying pan (preferably nonstick or cast-iron)

⅓-cup (80-ml) measuring cup or portion scoop

Preheat the oven to 400°F (200°C, or gas mark 6). Line a baking tray with parchment paper.

Make the Cumin-Roasted Vegetables: While the oven heats up, combine the broccoli, bell pepper, squash, and onion in a large mixing bowl with olive oil, cumin, cumin seeds (if using), salt, and a few grinds of black pepper. Toss well to combine and coat each piece with the seasonings. Transfer to the baking tray and pop into the oven with a timer set for 25 minutes.

Make the Turnip Hash Browns: While the veggies cook, crack the egg into a large mixing bowl and whisk with ⅛ teaspoon each of salt and pepper. Peel the turnips and grate on a box grater. Feel free to shred with the grating attachment of a food processor if you have one available! Add the turnips to the egg and stir to ensure all pieces of turnip get coated in egg.

Heat a frying pan over medium-high heat until a drop of water sizzles upon contact. Melt 1 tablespoon (14 g) of the fat of your choice until it runs freely around the pan but is not smoking. Drop ⅓ cup (80 ml) of the turnip-egg mixture into the pan, leaving about 1-inch (2.5-cm) between the piles. Flatten slightly and cook for 4 to 5 minutes per side until edges are starting to get crispy and they are lightly browned in entirety. Remove from the pan to a plate and repeat process, wiping out pan in between. Depending on the size of the frying pan, you may need a little additional fat.

If you finish the hash browns before the vegetables are finished cooking, place them in the oven on an oven-safe plate to keep warm.

Make the yogurt sauce: In a small mixing bowl, combine the yogurt and chili powder. Season to taste with salt. Set aside.

Once vegetables have been removed from oven and hash browns are done, divide the hash browns among four plates. Top with one-quarter of the roasted vegetables and about 2 tablespoons (30 ml) of sauce. Yumarific!

Nutritional Information: Calories: 184 – Protein: 6.2 g – Fat: 11.5 g – Carbs: 16.7 g – Fiber: 3.9 g – Net carbs: 12.5 g – Sodium: 382 mg – Potassium: 569 mg

Asparagus and Goat Cheese Frittata with Fresh Herb Salad

Goat cheese and asparagus combine to make this one quick and delicious meal. The tart creaminess of the goat cheese pairs perfectly with the mellow-flavored, crisp-tender asparagus, and the herb salad brings the combination to the next level of delicious and nutritious. My clients are always excited when this turns up on the menu. The best part is that it takes almost no time to throw together!

Total time: 20 minutes   **Yield:** 1 frittata (2 servings)

Frittata

3 eggs

1 cup chopped fresh asparagus (about 10 ounces [280 g] spears trimmed)

¼ cup (40 g) small-dice onion

Salt and black pepper

1 tablespoon (15 ml) extra-virgin olive oil

¼ cup (38 g) crumbled goat cheese

Herb Salad

2 cups (110 g) mixed baby greens

1 cup (60 g) fresh parsley leaves

¼ cup (24 g) fresh mint leaves, torn

¼ cup (12 g) fresh basil leaves, torn

Zest and juice of 1 lemon

1 tablespoon (15 ml) extra-virgin olive oil

Salt and black pepper

Accessories needed:

2 medium mixing bowls

Small 8- to 9-inch (20- to 23-inch) frying pan

Preheat the oven to 350°F (175°C, or gas mark 4).

Make the frittata: Whisk together eggs, asparagus, onion, salt, and pepper in a medium mixing bowl. Heat the oil in a small frying pan over medium-high heat, and once the oil runs freely around the pan, pour in the egg mixture. *Do not stir.* Sprinkle the goat cheese all over the top and cook for 4 minutes, allowing to set.

Transfer the entire pan into the warmed oven and cook for 11 to 12 minutes, until the top is lightly browned and no longer jiggly. Using an oven mitt, potholder, or DRY kitchen towel, remove the pan from the oven and set aside on the stovetop to cool.

Make the salad: Combine mixed baby greens, fresh herbs, and lemon zest in a mixing bowl. Toss to evenly distribute the zest among the leaves, then add lemon juice and olive oil and toss again to coat. Season with salt and pepper.

Divide frittata among 2 plates and serve with salad alongside.

Nutritional Information: Calories: 351 – Protein: 18.1 g – Fat: 27.3 g – Carbs: 10.8 g – Fiber: 6.8 g – Net carbs: 4 g – Sodium: 273 mg – Potassium: 622 mg

Poultry Mains

Winner winner, chicken dinner! And turkey, too . . . Poultry is a worldwide favorite, and with good reason. It's affordable, easy to find, and sparkles whether simple or tossed in a sauce!

You can taste shades of my own mother's cooking in the Clean Classic Chicken Cacciatore (page 132), and I highly recommend the Bacon-Wrapped Rosemary Chicken & Creamed Baby Greens (page 135) for a super-satisfying yet simple-to-make dinner perfect for entertaining.

Lemon Thyme Roasted Chicken Thighs

Here's roast chicken without the hour-and-a-half wait—and some crispy skin action, too. Thyme has a plant compound called thymol that has proven antibiotic, antifungal, and antiviral properties. You'll be giving your immune system a boost while enjoying a very homey meal.

Total time: 35 minutes   **Yield:** 4 to 6 servings (1 to 2 chicken thighs each)

2 pounds (910 g) bone-in and skin-on chicken thighs

2 tablespoons (30 ml) extra-virgin olive oil

1 tablespoon (2 g) fresh lemon thyme or 1 teaspoon dried lemon thyme

Salt and black pepper (Omnivore Limone blend is my favorite to substitute here!)

Accessories needed:

Baking tray

Parchment paper

Preheat the oven to 400°F (200°C, or gas mark 6). Line baking tray with parchment paper.

Place the chicken on the parchment. Drizzle with olive oil, sprinkle with lemon thyme, and season with salt and pepper. Make sure the oil and herbs cover each piece before turning them skin-side down and placing in the oven.

Bake for 20 minutes and flip. Bake for 10 minutes until cooked through—check for an internal temperature of 165°F (74°C). Remove from the oven, cool slightly, and eat!

Nutritional Information (based on 5 servings): Calories: 405 – Protein: 30 g – Fat: 32 g – Carbs: 0 g – Fiber: 0 g – Net carbs: 0 g – Sodium: 274 mg – Potassium: 348 mg

Clean Classic Chicken Cacciatore

Just like mom used to make—but healthier! The chicken delivers protein and the tomatoes provide vitamins A and C, plus the cancer-fighting, heart-protective antioxidant lycopene. This dish was one of my favorites growing up, but I flipped the script to make it just a little heartier while still feeling light. It's such a fall-off-the-bone, winner chicken dinner, especially when accompanied by fresh zucchini noodles or even traditional pasta aglio e olio.

Total time: 1 hour 15 minutes **Yield:** 4 servings

4 bone-in and skin-on chicken thighs

4 drumsticks

Salt and black pepper

1 tablespoon (15 ml) extra-virgin olive oil

1 cup (115 g) sliced onion

4 stalks celery chopped width-ways into ¼-inch (6-mm) pieces

2 cloves garlic, crushed

1 can (14.5 ounces, or 411 g) diced tomatoes

1 can (8 ounces, or 225 g) tomato sauce

¼ teaspoon salt

1 teaspoon dried oregano

2 bay leaves

⅓ cup (80 ml) dry white wine

Accessory needed:

Large skillet with a lid

Season the chicken with salt and pepper all over.

Heat a large skillet over medium heat until a drop of water sizzles upon hitting and add olive oil. Swirl the oil to cover the pan and brown the chicken on all sides, starting with skin-side down first. You may have to do this in batches—start with the thighs. Remove browned chicken and set aside on a plate.

Remove half of the rendered fat that has gathered in the pan and then add the onion, celery, and garlic. Cook, stirring frequently, until the onions and celery are getting soft but not brown, about 5 minutes. Stir in the tomatoes, tomato sauce, salt, oregano, and bay leaves. Simmer for 2 to 3 minutes. Return the chicken to pan, nestling it into the sauce.

Cover and simmer for 30 minutes. Add the white wine and cook uncovered for 10 minutes. Remove the bay leaves. Divide among four plates and ladle ½ cup (120 ml) of sauce over chicken when serving.

Nutritional Information: Calories: 443 – Protein: 30 g – Fat: 30 g – Carbs: 11 g – Fiber: 3.8 g – Net carbs: 7.2 g – Sodium: 630 mg – Potassium: 802 mg

Bacon-Wrapped Rosemary Chicken & Creamed Baby Greens

Looking for soul-warming comfort food that will satisfy all your nutritional needs?
Look no further! This chicken is out-of-this-world delicious, especially in combination
with these super quick, super healthy greens.

Total time: 45 minutes   **Yield:** 4 servings

Bacon-Wrapped Rosemary Chicken

2 (6–8 ounces, or 168–225 g each) chicken breasts

Salt and black pepper

2 rosemary spears

4 slices thinner-cut bacon

Creamed Baby Greens

1 tablespoon (15 ml) extra-virgin olive oil

¼ cup (40 g) chopped onion

¼ teaspoon salt

10 ounces (280 g) baby leafy greens (spinach, kale, power blend, any of 'em!)

¼ cup (60 ml) heavy cream

2 ounces (55 g) cream cheese, broken into little pieces

Pinch nutmeg (optional)

Accessories needed:

Meat tenderizer or bottle

Oven-safe frying pan

Medium saucepan

Preheat the oven to 400°F (200°C, or gas mark 6).

Make the chicken: Place one chicken breast between two pieces of plastic wrap (or one long piece folded over) and use a meat tenderizer or bottle to pound to ½-inch (1cm) thickness. Set aside on a plate and repeat process with second breast. Season on both sides with salt and pepper.

Place a rosemary spear on one side of flattened breast and roll tightly. Once it is in a cylindrical shape, start winding bacon slices around in a spiral fashion about 1 inch (2.5 cm) from end, overlapping edges slightly. You should use 2 slices per breast.

Once both breasts have been covered in bacon, heat an oven-safe pan over medium-high heat until a droplet of water sizzles. Place both breasts in the pan, bacon ends–side down first. Brown on all sides, turning every 2 to 3 minutes, and then transfer entire pan directly to oven for 15 minutes.

Remember to use an oven mitt to remove the pan from oven! Let the meat rest for 5 minutes before slicing into ½-inch (1cm) thick rounds. Remove woody stem pieces of rosemary before eating.

Make the greens: Heat oil in a medium saucepan over medium-high heat until it swirls quickly around the pan. Add the onion and salt and sauté for 2 minutes, until the edges start to brown. Stir in the greens until they are just about completely wilted but still bright in color, about 30 seconds. Pour in the heavy cream, add the cream cheese, and sprinkle in nutmeg (if using). Lower the heat to medium-low and stir until cream cheese is completely melted.

Nutritional Information: Calories: 388 – Protein: 29.4 g – Fat: 28 g – Carbs: 5.3 g – Fiber: 2 g – Net carbs: 3.3 g – Sodium: 480 mg – Potassium: 834 mg

Turkey-Mushroom Meatloaf Muffins

Meatloaf is so much better when it's fun-sized! These little babies can be enjoyed as a high-protein snack or as part of a larger meal. I often pair them with the Gingery Green Beans from the Miso-Glazed Tofu recipe (page 116).

Total time: 23 minutes   **Yield:** 4 servings (3 pieces per serving)

1½ pounds (680 g) ground turkey

5 ounces (140 g) shiitake or button mushrooms, chopped finely

¼ cup (40 g) finely chopped onion

2 tablespoons (32 g) tomato paste

1 tablespoon (15 ml) coconut aminos

½ teaspoon garlic powder

1 egg

Salt and black pepper

Cooking spray or oil for greasing muffin tin

Accessories needed:

Mixing bowl

12-well muffin tin

Place all ingredients apart from cooking spray in a mixing bowl and combine thoroughly until the mixture is homogenous.

Grease the muffin tin with cooking spray—I prefer olive or avocado oil spray. Divide the turkey mixture among the wells. Bake for 20 minutes until firm and lightly browned on top. Remove from the oven and enjoy!

Nutritional Information: Calories: 350 – Protein: 32 g – Fat: 23 g – Carbs: 5.9 g – Fiber: 1.4 g – Net carbs: 4.5 g – Sodium: 185 mg – Potassium: 569 mg

Sticky Orange Chicken & Greens "On Fire"

This chicken is how I like life to be—sweet and spicy and overall good for you! Paired with my take on my favorite greens dish in the world, the Thai Pak Boong Fai Deng, or "Morning Glory in Flames," and you have an utterly, ridiculously, scrumptiously delicious and nutritious combo that will also kick you in the pants spice-wise. Don't worry—you can adjust the heat.

Total time: 40 minutes   **Yield:** 2 servings

Sticky Orange Chicken

1 teaspoon baking soda (bicarbonate of soda)

1 tablespoon (9 g) plus ½ teaspoon arrowroot or cornstarch, divided

Salt and black pepper

1 pound (455 g) boneless, skinless chicken breast, chopped into 1-inch (2.5-cm) pieces

Zest and juice of 1 pound (455 g) of oranges or clementines

3 tablespoons (45 ml) rice wine vinegar

2 tablespoons (30 ml) coconut aminos

½ teaspoon ground ginger

2 tablespoons (30 ml) avocado oil

1 tablespoon (10 g) minced garlic

1 tablespoon (6 g) minced fresh ginger

¼ teaspoon crushed red pepper flakes

Greens on Fire

2 tablespoons (30 ml) coconut aminos or tamari

1 tablespoon (10 g) brown sugar substitute, brown sugar, coconut sugar, or palm sugar

¼ cup (60 ml) water

2 tablespoons (30 ml) avocado oil

2 cloves garlic, crushed

1–2 Thai bird's eye chile peppers, bruised and chopped in half (optional)

1½–2 pounds (680–910 g) Morning Glory, aka Ong Choy or Water Spinach (you can substitute bok choy or baby bok choy if you can't find ong choy), chopped into 2- to 3-inch (5 to 7.5 cm) pieces

Accessories needed:

Medium mixing bowl

Large frying pan, ideally nonstick

Air fryer makes this really easy, but not necessary

Baking tray

Parchment paper

Wire cooling rack

Cooking spray

Large frying pan or wok

Make the chicken: Preheat the oven to 425°F (220°C, or gas mark 6). Line the baking tray with parchment paper before placing wire rack on top. Spray the rack with cooking spray (I use avocado).

In the mixing bowl, combine baking soda, 1 tablespoon (9 g) arrowroot and a pinch each of salt and pepper. Pat the chicken as dry as possible with paper towels and toss in the powdery mixture. Place the chicken in a single layer on the wire rack and pop into the oven for 15 to 20 minutes, until it is cooked through and feels slightly dry and crispy on the outside.

Make the orange sauce: Meanwhile, prepare the orange sauce. In a small bowl, combine the juice, vinegar, coconut aminos, zest, ground ginger, and ½ teaspoon of arrowroot. Whisk well until no starch residue is left at the bottom of the bowl. Set aside.

In the large frying pan, heat the avocado oil until it runs freely around the pan and add the garlic, fresh ginger, and red pepper flakes with a teeny pinch of salt. Sauté until fragrant but not burning and quickly pour in the juice-vinegar mixture, whisking constantly and quickly while the sauce thickens, just a couple of minutes.

Remove the chicken from the oven and transfer directly into the sauce to coat. Garnish with fresh orange segments.

Make the greens: Whisk together the coconut aminos, brown sugar or substitute, and water in a small bowl and set aside.

Over high/medium-high heat, warm the frying pan and add the avocado oil. Once it flows freely around the pan, add the garlic and Thai chili peppers (if using), cooking until fragrant, about 30 seconds. Add the greens and quickly stir-fry so that they all become bright green and start wilting. Pour in the sugar-liquid mixture and stir through quickly. The greens will steam, leaving very little liquid left in the pan that isn't coming out of the greens themselves. Remove from the heat, remove chili and garlic, and enjoy alongside the orange chicken.

Nutritional Information: Calories: 504 – Protein: 11 g – Fat: 15 g – Carbs: 25 g – Fiber: 7.5 g – Net carbs: 17.5 g – Sodium: 716 mg – Potassium: 1872 mg

Lemon Basil Chicken Tenders & Tapenade Rice

Kids love this chicken, and it gets dressed up with one of my favorite easy Italian sides of rice salad, but with serious shortcuts! You can use regular cooked rice here if you so desire—it will add to the cooking time. I prefer using shirataki rice, which is pretty much ALL fiber, which feeds your gut and suits a protein-sparing modified fast with no issue. Plus, it's ridiculously quick to prepare. The recipe calls for cooking the chicken in the oven but making it in a grill pan or regular frying pan works fine, too.

Total time: 25 minutes   **Yield:** 2 servings

Lemon Basil Chicken

8 ounces (225 g) boneless, skinless chicken breast OR chicken breast tenderloins

1 tablespoon (15 ml) extra-virgin olive oil

Zest and juice of 1 lemon

2 tablespoons (6 g) finely chopped fresh basil

Salt and black pepper

Tapenade Rice

1 packet (8 ounces, or 225 g) rinsed and drained shirataki rice (such as Miracle Rice) or 1 cup (186 g) prepared white or brown rice

3 tablespoons (60 g) prepared olive tapenade (such as Divina)

Accessories needed:

Baking tray

Parchment paper

Mixing bowl

Small frying pan

Preheat the oven to 425°F (220°C, or gas mark 6). Line a baking tray with parchment paper.

Make the chicken: In the mixing bowl, combine the chicken tenders, olive oil, lemon zest, basil, and salt and pepper to taste. Toss well to coat. Transfer to a parchment paper lined baking tray in a single layer and spritz with half of the lemon juice just before placing into the oven. Bake for 10 to 15 minutes until cooked through. Remove and drizzle with remaining lemon juice to make it extra lemony!

Make the rice: Heat the frying pan over medium-high heat. Add the shirataki rice and dry fry for 5 minutes to get as much moisture out as possible. You will know when it's done when the rice becomes opaque and pieces start to jump out of the pan! Remove from the heat and stir in the tapenade. It's that easy!

For regular rice, you do not even need to heat it up. Just combine the tapenade with the cooked and cooled rice. An added benefit? Cooked and cooled rice has more resistant starch than freshly cooked rice! That gives it prebiotic qualities, making your gut happy, and creating a lower glycemic response when you eat it. How awesome is that!?

Nutritional Information: Calories: 282 – Protein: 26.6 g – Fat: 17.1 g – Carbs: 5.5 g – Fiber: 0.9 g – Net carbs: 4.6 g – Sodium: 257 mg – Potassium: 449 mg

Beef, Pork, and Lamb Mains

There's nothing that I find more grounding and filling than a well-prepared meat-based dish, especially accompanied by the perfect veggie side or power-packed sauce. They make me feel like I have ticked all of my macronutrient boxes in one fell swoop! Protein? Super check! Fat? Yep! Low-glycemic carbohydrates? You know it!

Slightly sweet Lean Lemongrass Pork Skewers & Purple Sesame Slaw (page 146) is a delicious budget-friendly option that makes for AMAZING leftover lunch the next day. And if you want to make ahead and freeze, try the Perfect Protein-Packed Stuffed Peppers (page 149). They'll go faster than you can say the recipe name ten times fast!

Pan-Fried Flank Steak & Best Blender Chimichurri

Flank steak is such a versatile protein. It marinates and cooks quickly, is a great source of lean protein, and provides an amazing vehicle for this super-nutritious, detoxifying, under-appreciated herbaceous condiment! This chimichurri will inspire you, and while it's perfect on the steak, it pairs well with just about every other protein you can imagine, too.

Total time: 23 minutes   **Yield:** 4 servings

1 pound (455 g) flank steak

2 tablespoons (30 ml) Worcestershire sauce or coconut aminos

¼ teaspoon fine salt

⅛ teaspoon freshly ground black pepper

½ teaspoon avocado oil, if needed

Accessories needed:

Shallow dish

Nonstick or cast-iron frying pan

In a shallow dish, marinate steak with Worcestershire sauce, salt, and pepper for 10 minutes. Heat a frying pan over high heat until a droplet of water sizzles and evaporates within seconds. If using cast-iron, brush ½ teaspoon oil into pan. Place the steak in the pan and cook for 3 to 4 minutes on each side. Remove from the pan and move to a plate. Cover with foil and let rest while the chimichurri is being prepared.

1 cup (65 g) packed fresh flat-leaf parsley

1 cup (16 g) loosely packed fresh cilantro leaves

2 tablespoons (8 g) fresh dill

1 tablespoon (4 g) fresh oregano

¼ cup (38 g) sweet bell pepper

2 green onions

2–3 small to medium cloves garlic

Pinch salt

Pinch ground cumin

⅓ cup (80 ml) extra-virgin olive oil

¼ cup (60 ml) red wine vinegar (you can use lemon juice or white or white wine vinegar if that's all you have)

Accessory needed:

Blender

Best Blender Chimichurri

Total time: 5 minutes
Yield: 12 servings (2 tablespoons [24 g] each)

Put it all in a blender and blend away until it looks uniform in bright green color. Slather on steak and enjoy! Store in an airtight container for up to 2 weeks.

Nutritional Information: Calories: 246 – Protein: 24.2 g – Fat: 14.7 g – Carbs: 2.6 g – Fiber: .3 g – Net carbs: 2.3 g – Sodium: 367 mg – Potassium: 472 mg

Quick Korean-Flavored Marinated Beef & Kimchi Kale Fried Rice

Korean cuisine is one of my favorites, but because I am allergic to gluten and also sugar free, I can typically only enjoy it prepared at home or by one of my Korean cousins. This recipe is scrumptious and a love-and-nutrient-filled homage to deliciousness.

Total time: 1 hour, 10 minutes   **Yield:** 4 servings

Korean Marinated Beef

1 pound (455 g) very thinly sliced ribeye or tenderloin (Ask your butcher for help with this or freeze the meat *slightly* to get it firm and slice as thinly as possible with a very sharp knife.)

1 tablespoon (15 ml) toasted sesame oil

¼ cup (28 g) thinly sliced onion

3 green onions, finely chopped

1 tablespoon (8 g) toasted white sesame seeds

Gochujang Korean hot sauce (optional)

Marinade

2 tablespoons (30 ml) toasted sesame oil

¼ cup (60 ml) tamari or coconut aminos

1 tablespoon (10 g) minced garlic

¼ teaspoon gochugaru, Korean chili flakes, or crushed red pepper flakes

2 tablespoons (20 g) brown sugar substitute (I like Lakanto golden or Sukrin gold)

1 tablespoon (15 ml) toasted sesame oil

Freshly ground black pepper

Kimchi Kale Fried Rice

1 tablespoon (15 ml) avocado oil

1 tablespoon (15 ml) plus 1 teaspoon toasted sesame oil

2 cups (226 g) raw cauliflower rice OR regular white, brown, or shirataki rice

½ cup (34 g) packed torn kale

½ cup (120 g) chopped kimchi

Salt

½ tablespoon (8 ml) gochujang or sriracha

½ tablespoon (8 ml) tamari

1 egg

2 tablespoons (16 g) toasted white sesame seeds

Accessories needed:

Gallon resealable plastic bag

Blender

Nonstick frying pan or wok

Tongs

Prepare the beef and marinade: Place the beef and onion into the resealable plastic bag. Combine all the marinade ingredients in the blender and process until well combined. Pour over the beef, squeeze as much air as you can out of the bag, and let chill in the fridge for 30 minutes while you make the fried rice.

Make the rice: Add the avocado oil and 1 teaspoon of toasted sesame oil to the pan over medium-high heat. Once it swirls easily around the pan, add the cauliflower rice and kale with a pinch of salt and stir-fry until the kale is bright green and starting to wilt, about 3 minutes. Add in the kimchi with its juice, gochujang, and tamari. Cook, stirring frequently, until the liquid has just about completely evaporated.

Create a well in the middle of the pan by pushing the fried rice off to the sides and add the remaining tablespoon of sesame oil. Crack in the egg, breaking the yolk, and sprinkle a pinch of salt on top. Allow to cook until no longer runny with the bottom turning brown, crispy, and starting to sputter. Remove from the heat and use cooking spoon or spatula to break up the egg and stir into the rest of the rice. Stir in the sesame seeds for extra texture.

Make the Korean marinated beef: Once the fried rice is done, remove beef from fridge. Warm 1 tablespoon (15 ml) of the toasted sesame oil in the frying pan or wok over medium-high heat until it flows freely around the pan. Using tongs, transfer half of the meat-and-onion mixture to the pan, allowing as much liquid to drain back into the bag as possible. Stir-fry the beef until just cooked and move to a plate or bowl, covering with foil while you repeat the process for the second half of the beef.

Once all the beef is cooked, pour the marinade left in the bag into the still-hot pan and reduce by half before pouring over the beef for extra yum-yum flavor! Garnish with green onions and sesame seeds and spice up with fermented gluten-free gochujang Korean hot sauce (if using)! SO GOOD!

Nutritional Information: Calories: 536 – Protein: 26.8 g – Fat: 41 g – Carbs: 16.8 g – Fiber: 2.8 g – Net carbs: 14 g – Sodium: 635 mg – Potassium: 580 mg

Lean Lemongrass Pork Skewers & Purple Sesame Slaw

Grilled lemongrass pork skewers are one of my favorite things of all time! With only a handful of ingredients, they are ridiculously easy to make—and highly nutritious. This dish is filled with fiber, antioxidants, and B vitamins. It's absolutely gorgeous with a simple sesame slaw, too.

Total time: 45 minutes   **Yield:** 4 servings

Skewers

1 pound (455 g) pork sirloin or shoulder steak

2 tablespoons (18 g) coconut sugar or granulated monk fruit sweetener

1 stalk lemongrass, white parts only, chopped

2 tablespoons (30 ml) coconut aminos or tamari

2 tablespoons (30 ml) fish sauce

1 tablespoon (15 ml) avocado oil

Slaw

3 tablespoons (45 ml) rice wine vinegar

1½ tablespoons (25 ml) avocado oil

½ tablespoon (8 ml) sesame oil

1 teaspoon coconut aminos

Salt and black pepper

4 cups (280 g) finely shredded red cabbage

1 purple carrot, julienned

2 green onions, finely chopped on the bias

1 tablespoon (8 g) toasted white sesame seeds

Accessories needed:

Baking tray

Parchment paper

Medium and large mixing bowls

Blender or food processor

3-inch (7.5 cm) skewers

Grill pan or frying pan

Pro-tip:

Add the oil straight to the marinade so the skewers don't stick to the grill.

Preheat the oven to 400°F (200°C, or gas mark 6). Line a baking tray with parchment paper.

Make the skewers: Slice the pork thinly into 2- to 3-inch (5 to 7.5 cm) pieces. Place into a medium mixing bowl.

Combine the sweetener, lemongrass, coconut aminos, fish sauce, and avocado oil in a blender and process until smooth. Pour over the pork and mix well to coat all the pieces. Thread each piece onto a skewer and replace in bowl to soak up as much marinade as possible.

Heat a grill pan over medium-high heat. When a drop of water sizzles on contact, lay the skewers on the pan, leaving plenty of room in between to not crowd the pan. You may have to cook these in 2 to 3 batches. Cook for about 2 minutes per side, until some nice brown grill marks appear. Transfer to the baking tray. Once all skewers have been marked, place the tray in the oven for 10 minutes.

Make the slaw: While the skewers cook, whisk together the rice wine vinegar, avocado oil, sesame oil, and coconut aminos in a large mixing bowl. Taste and adjust seasoning with salt and pepper. Add the cabbage, carrot, and green onions. Massage the dressing through. The volume of the vegetables will decrease significantly. Stir in the sesame seeds and season to taste.

Remove the skewers from the oven. Allow to cool just slightly, so you can touch the skewers. Serve 3 to 4 of the skewers alongside one-quarter of the slaw.

Nutritional Information: Calories: 388 – Protein: 35.8 g – Fat: 20 g – Carbs: 16.4 g – Fiber: 2.6 g – Net carbs: 14.4 g – Sodium: 972 mg – Potassium: 749 mg

Creamy Sausage-Stuffed Jalapeños

These peppers come together quickly and easily, and they are usually consumed the same way. The only difficult part of this recipe is stopping at a serving size, even though the perfectly delicious combination of protein, fat, and spices will satisfy your physical hunger with only a few pieces.

Total time: 35 minutes   **Yield:** 10 servings (4 pepper halves per serving)

1–1¼ pounds (455–570 g) mild Italian sausage, bulk or casings removed

1 package (8 ounces, or 225g) cream cheese

½ cup (40 g) grated Parmesan

20 fresh jalapeño peppers

Accessories needed:

Baking tray

Parchment paper

Large skillet

Gloves

Small spoon

Preheat the oven to 375°F (190°C, or gas mark 5). Line a baking tray with parchment paper.

Heat a large skillet over medium-high heat. Crumble and sauté the sausage until fully cooked, about 10 minutes, constantly breaking up the sausage into smaller and smaller bits. Once it is fully cooked, reduce the heat to medium and add cream cheese, stirring often as you melt it completely. Once the cream cheese is fully combined with the sausage, remove from the heat and stir through Parmesan until well combined. Set aside to cool.

Best done wearing gloves: Cut the jalapeños in half lengthwise and use a spoon to scoop out the seeds and white membrane. Place them on the baking tray and stuff each pepper with the sausage-cheese mixture until it is all gone.

Bake for 15 to 20 minutes. The jalapeños lose their bite when they are cooked until soft—that is when you want to take them out of the oven. Cool for a few minutes and enjoy.

Nutritional Information: Calories: 287 – Protein: 10 g – Fat: 26 g – Carbs: 4 g – Fiber: .8 g – Net carbs: 3.2 g – Sodium: 77 mg – Potassium: 239 mg

Perfect Stuffed Peppers

All goodness stuffed into an edible container. What could be better?

Total time: 35 minutes   **Yield:** 4 servings

4 medium green peppers

1 pound (450 g) sweet Italian sausage

3 cups (320 g) riced cauliflower

¼ cup (28 g) flax meal

½ cup (80 g) minced onion

1 cup (245 g) low sugar tomato sauce (I used Rao's marinara), divided

1 cup (240 ml) water

Accessories needed:

Large mixing bowl

Electric pressure cooker (you can do this on the stove or oven, it just takes longer)

Core and deseed the peppers and set aside.

In a large mixing bowl, combine sausage, cauliflower, flax meal, onion, and ½ cup (122 g) of the tomato sauce. Combine well with your hands or a fork and then divide evenly among the hollowed-out peppers.

Place the peppers stuffing side up in the pressure cooker and pour the remaining ½ cup (122 g) of sauce and the water into the bottom of the pot.

Secure the lid and set to high pressure for 15 minutes. Once finished, you can either wait for pressure to release gradually, or very carefully flip the switch to vent quickly—the steam is very hot so use caution.

If using a stove instead of a pressure cooker, add 2 cups (480 ml) of water to a pot and cook, covered, for 45 minutes over medium heat with the lid slightly ajar. In the oven, opt for cutting the peppers in half vertically and laying in a baking dish stuffing side up with just 1 cup (240 ml) of water. Cover with foil and bake for 60 minutes at 375°F (190°C or gas mark 5).

Nutritional Information: Calories: 440 – Protein: 22 g - Fat: 15 g – Carbs: 14 g - Fiber: 4 g – Net carbs: 10 g – Sodium: 864 mg – Potassium: 471 mg

Dijon Pork Tenderloin & Beet and Citrus Salad

Two kinds of beta-carotene-rich beets and three kinds of vitamin C–abundant citrus provide the perfect naturally sweet, antioxidant, and super-colorful foil to the earthier, lean, mustardy pork tenderloin. This dish tastes as elegant as it looks and would be as much welcomed at a casual dinner as a lovely dinner party.

Total time: 45 minutes   **Yield:** 4 servings

Pork

1 pound (455 g) pork tenderloin

Salt and black pepper

2 tablespoons (30 g) Dijon mustard, divided

1 tablespoon (15 ml) avocado oil

Broth, if needed

Salad

1 orange (zested, then peeled and sliced into rounds)

1 grapefruit (zested, then peeled and sliced into rounds)

Zest and juice of 1 lemon

2 tablespoons (30 ml) extra-virgin olive oil

1 teaspoon minced garlic

½ pound (225 g) red beets (2 medium beets)

1 medium yellow beet

1 cup (60 g) loosely packed fresh parsley leaves

2 tablespoons (20 g) thinly sliced shallot

1 teaspoon coriander seeds

Accessories needed:

Frying pan

Medium mixing bowl

Mandoline or grating attachment with food processor

Pie tin

Meat thermometer

Preheat the oven to 400°F (200°C, or gas mark 6).

Trim the silver skin off the pork tenderloin and season all over with salt and pepper. Coat tenderloin with 1 tablespoon (15 g) Dijon mustard. Heat the frying pan over medium-high heat until a drop of water sizzles immediately upon being dropped in. Add the avocado oil to the pan and heat until it runs freely around the pan. Place tenderloin in the pan and cook for 1 to 2 minutes per side, until evenly browned all over. Transfer to oven directly in the pan for 15 minutes.

While that cooks, combine the zest of the citrus, lemon juice, any juice collected when slicing grapefruit and orange, olive oil, and garlic in the mixing bowl and whisk together. Season to taste with salt and pepper.

Peel and julienne the beets with a mandoline or grating attachment of a food processor. Add to the dressing, along with the parsley, shallots, and citrus rounds. Mix well.

Place the coriander seeds in the pie tin and toast in the oven for 5 minutes. Add to the beet-citrus mixture.

The meat should be ready at this time, with an internal temperature of 165°F (74°C). Using an oven mitt, take the pan out of the oven and let stand, covered, for 10 minutes.

Remove the tenderloin from the pan and whisk remaining tablespoon of Dijon mustard into the pan juices. You can add a splash of bone broth (chicken or pork) to thin out the sauce slightly.

Thinly slice the pork into medallions. Divide the salad among four plates and arrange one-quarter of the pork medallions alongside. Drizzle with pan sauce.

Nutritional Information: Calories: 321 – Protein: 26 g – Fat: 15 g – Carbs: 22 g – Fiber: 5.1 g – Net carbs: 169 g – Sodium: 332 mg – Potassium: 971 mg

Balsamic Lamb Chops and Loaded Quinoa Tabbouleh

Lamb is a dinner option many people forget about, but it is such a wonderful source of protein, packed with iron, and cooks up quickly. This combination makes particularly amazing leftovers for lunch the following day. Using a rice cooker for the quinoa is a revolutionizing technique that will make your life so much easier, but don't worry if you don't have one. It's easy to do on the stovetop as well.

Total time: 45 minutes   **Yield:** 4 servings

Quinoa

1 cup (173 g) quinoa

2 cups (475 ml) water

Pinch salt

½ cup (70 g) peeled and chopped cucumbers

½ cup (62 g) chopped tomato

¼ cup (56 g) crumbled feta cheese

½ cup (30 g) loosely packed fresh parsley

¼ cup (60 ml) extra-virgin olive oil

¼ cup (60 ml) lemon juice

Zest of 1 lemon

Salt and black pepper

Lamb

4 regular lamb chops or 8 baby lamb chops

Salt and black pepper

1 teaspoon chopped rosemary

1 teaspoon thyme leaves

Zest of 1 lemon

1 tablespoon (15 ml) extra-virgin olive oil

½ cup (120 ml) balsamic vinegar

Accessories needed:

Fine-mesh strainer

Rice cooker OR small saucepan with lid

Large mixing bowl

Frying pan

**Balsamic Lamb Chops and Loaded
Quinoa Tabbouleh** (continued from page 152)

Make the quinoa: Rinse the quinoa in a fine-mesh strainer until the water runs clear. Transfer to a rice cooker with 2 cups (475 ml) of water and a pinch of salt and press cook. If you are using the stovetop, transfer to a small saucepan after rinsing and add water and salt. Bring to a boil over medium-high heat. Reduce the heat to low and simmer, covered, until all the water is absorbed, about 20 minutes. Remove from the heat and transfer to a large mixing bowl to cool.

Make the lamb: While the quinoa is cooking, season the lamb chops with salt, pepper, rosemary, thyme, and lemon zest. Heat the oil in the frying pan over medium-high heat until it shimmers and flows easily around the pan. Add the lamb chops and cook for 4 minutes per side for regular lamb chops, 2 minutes per side for baby lamb chops. If you use baby lamb chops, you may need to do this in 2 batches.

When the lamb is browned on each side and feels like the pad of your thumb to the touch—firm with a little give—it is medium rare and ready to be transferred to a waiting plate. Alternatively, you can check the internal temperature with a meat thermometer and are looking for 135°F to 140°F (57°C to 60°C). Once on the plate, cover with aluminum foil.

Pour the balsamic vinegar into the lamb pan, scraping any cooked bits off the bottom of the pan. Lower the heat to medium-low and reduce by a third. The sauce should be thicker but not syrupy. Remove from the heat.

By this time, the quinoa should be finished cooking and be in the cooling stage. Once it is only warm to the touch—not hot—you can add the remainder of the tabbouleh ingredients and mix well.

Return the balsamic sauce to the stove over low heat, just to warm. Stir any juices that have been released on the plate to the sauce and whisk slightly. Return the lamb to the pan and flip to coat in the warm sauce.

Divide the tabbouleh onto 4 plates and place a lamb chop (or two!) to the side. Drizzle the lamb with the pan sauce and dig in!

Nutritional Information: Calories 551 – Protein: 36.1 g – Fat: 27.9 g – Carbs: 39.6 g – Fiber: 4.9 g – Net carbs: 34.7 g – Sodium: 225 mg – Potassium: 707 mg – Potassium: 211 mg

Fish Mains

Having grown up close to the ocean and lived and worked on boats for more than ten years, I have a passion for seafood and like to tell people that I'm half mermaid. Seafood is one of the quickest, easiest, and naturally leanest proteins to cook, and it is a phenomenal source of iron and iodine, among other nutrients.

Got fifteen minutes? Have Mediterranean Baked Shrimp (page 158) or Bright Coriander Roasted Salmon (page 160) on your table in that time, whipping up a quick salad while it cooks. Or take a little longer to treat yo'self with Italian Seared Tuna (page 159) and its slow-reducing Spicy Tomato Cream Sauce with steamed broccolini and your favorite noodles. The world is your oyster—pun intended!

Vibrant Veggie Shrimp Stir-Fry with Cashews & "Egg Roll" Fried Rice

This duo of dishes comes together so fast once they're prepped and provides a smorgasbord of vegetable heaven with a wide variety of colors, textures, and flavors. You could just as easily enjoy the recipes separately, but why would you?

Total time: 40 minutes   **Yield:** 2 servings

Stir-Fry

8 ounces (225 g) raw, peeled shrimp, 26–30 size or larger

Salt and black pepper

1 tablespoon (15 ml) neutral tasting oil (I like avocado.)

1 cup (71 g) broccoli florets, broken into bite-sized pieces

1 cup (75 g) snow peas, trimmed and de-threaded

1 tablespoon (6 g) minced fresh ginger

1 teaspoon minced garlic

½ cup (68 g) cashews

2 tablespoons (30 ml) coconut aminos or tamari

Egg Roll Fried Rice

1 tablespoon (15 ml) neutral flavored oil

½ cup (35 g) shredded green cabbage

½ cup (55 g) shredded carrot

2 green onions, divided into white and green parts, finely chopped

2 teaspoons (4 g) minced fresh ginger

1 teaspoon minced garlic

Salt

½ teaspoon sesame oil

1 cup (113 g) cauliflower rice or cooked white rice

1 egg

1 tablespoon (15 ml) coconut aminos or tamari

Accessory needed:

Frying pan or wok

Make the stir-fry: Season the shrimp lightly with salt and pepper. Heat the oil in a frying pan over high heat until it flows freely around the pan. Add the shrimp, broccoli, and snow peas. Cook for 2 minutes, stirring frequently. Add the ginger, garlic, and cashews. Incorporate well and cook for 2 to 3 minutes. By this time, the shrimp should be almost completely opaque, and the ginger and garlic will be fragrant and starting to brown.

Stir in the coconut aminos, which will steam through the vegetables and almost completely evaporate within 1 minute. Remove from the heat and transfer to a dish, covering to keep warm while you make the fried rice.

Make the rice: Rinse out the frying pan and return it to the stove over medium-high heat. When a drop of water sizzles instantly upon being dropped into the pan, add the oil. As soon as it shimmers, add the cabbage, carrot, white parts of the green onion, ginger, garlic, and a pinch of salt. Combine well and cook for 5 minutes, stirring frequently to prevent the garlic and ginger from browning. When the cabbage becomes soft and almost translucent, add the sesame oil and rice and cook for 3 minutes.

Make a well in the center of the mixture and crack the egg in, immediately breaking the yolk. Allow it to cook for about 30 seconds before blending it through the rest of the mixture. Finally, stir 1 tablespoon (15 ml) of coconut aminos through and remove from the heat.

Divide the stir-fry and fried rice between two plates. Garnish with the green parts of the green onions.

Nutritional Information: Calories: 536 – Protein: 28 g – Fat: 35 g – Carbs: 32 g – Fiber: 6.1 g – Net carbs: 25.9 g – Sodium: 1358 mg – Potassium: 932 mg

Mediterranean Baked Shrimp

It's in, it's out, it's gone! Baking shrimp is the fastest hack ever, and these little guys win rave reviews every time. The nutrient-packed oregano and thyme add flavor and zing.

Total time: 15 minutes   **Yield:** 3 to 4 servings (4 ounces [115 g] cooked shrimp per serving)

1 pound (455 g) raw, peeled, deveined, fresh or thawed shrimp

2 tablespoons (30 ml) extra-virgin olive oil

1 tablespoon (4 g) fresh oregano

½ tablespoon fresh thyme or lemon thyme

Zest of 1 lemon

Salt and black pepper

Accessories needed:

Baking tray

Parchment paper

Medium mixing bowl

Preheat the oven to 400°F (200°C, or gas mark 6). Line a baking tray with parchment paper.

In the medium mixing bowl, combine all of the ingredients and toss well to coat shrimp. Place in a single layer on the parchment paper and pop into the oven. Bake for 10 to 12 minutes, until the shrimp are firm and not looking translucent along the thickest part.

Remove from the oven and enjoy!

Nutritional Information: Calories: 199 – Protein: 21 g – Fat: 11 g – Carbs: 5 g – Fiber: 1.4 g – Net carbs: 3.6 g – Sodium: 857 mg – Potassium: 230 mg

Italian Seared Tuna & Spicy Tomato Cream Sauce

France meets Italy in this tuna and spicy tomato cream dish. It's a happy marriage that pairs so well with steamed green vegetables that it will make you an absolute star in the eyes of your dinner guests.

Total time: 35 minutes **Yield:** 2 servings

1 tablespoon (15 ml) plus
2 teaspoons (10 ml) extra-
virgin olive oil, divided

⅓ cup (55 g) finely
chopped onion

1 teaspoon minced garlic

Pinch salt

1 cup (240 ml) no-sugar
added prepared marinara or
arrabiata sauce

Pinch red pepper flakes
(optional)

2 tablespoons (30 ml)
balsamic vinegar

⅓ cup (80 ml) heavy cream

8-10 ounces (225–280 g)
fresh tuna

Salt and black pepper

1 teaspoon dried Italian
seasoning or herbs de Provence

Accessories needed:

Small saucepan

Nonstick frying pan

In a small saucepan over medium-high heat, combine the olive oil, garlic, onion, and salt. Cook for 3 to 5 minutes until the onions start to become translucent. Add the cup of prepared sauce, pepper flakes (if using), and balsamic vinegar. Lower the heat to medium and allow sauce to reduce by a third, simmering for about 10 minutes. Add the cream to the sauce and simmer for 20 minutes until it is nice and thick.

While the sauce cooks, drizzle 1 teaspoon olive oil over the tuna and rub over the entire piece(s). Season liberally with salt, pepper, and the Italian seasoning. Allow to sit at room temperature while the sauce is cooking so the center won't be ice cold when you go to eat it after searing!

About 5 minutes before the sauce is scheduled to be done, heat the nonstick frying pan over medium-high heat. It is ready to sear when a droplet of water sizzles and evaporates immediately upon contact.

Place the remaining teaspoon of oil in the pan and swirl around. Place in the tuna steak(s) and cook for 90 seconds before flipping and cooking for 90 seconds. This will give you the nice rare strip in the middle. If you prefer your tuna cooked through, increase the cooking time per side by 30 seconds to 1 minute.

Nutritional Information: Calories: 490 – Protein: 30 g – Fat: 33 g – Carbs: 17 g – Fiber: 3 g – Net carbs: 14 g – Sodium: 77 mg – Potassium: 812 mg

Bright Coriander Roasted Salmon

Salmon is one of the most nutritious foods on the planet and super quick to make. This yummy version goes particularly well with Everyman Tzatziki (page 64) and Amchoor Roasted Asparagus (page 182)!

Total time: 16 minutes   **Yield:** 2 servings

10 ounces (280 g) salmon

Salt and black pepper

2 teaspoons (10 ml) lemon juice

1 teaspoon extra-virgin olive oil

½ teaspoon ground coriander

½ teaspoon lemon zest

½ teaspoon coriander seeds

Accessories needed:

Pie tin or small baking tray

Parchment paper

Small mixing bowl

Preheat the oven to 425°F (220°C, or gas mark 6). Line a pie tin with parchment paper.

Place salmon on the parchment either in one piece or cut into 2 fillets. Season with salt and pepper. Set aside.

In a small mixing bowl, whisk together the lemon juice, olive oil, ground coriander, and lemon zest. Distribute evenly over the salmon, and then sprinkle the coriander seeds on top.

Pop into the oven and bake for 11 minutes. At this point, it will be cooked on the outside and still perfectly moist on the inside. Remove from the oven and enjoy!

Nutritional Information: Calories: 318 – Protein: 29 g – Fat: 21 g – Carbs: .8 g – Fiber: .5 g – Net carbs: .3 g – Sodium: 85 mg – Potassium: 532 mg

Sardine Fritters

Sardines are seriously underappreciated. Most days, I eat a can over the kitchen sink—honestly!—and I bring a can to every event I chef at. My assistants laugh at me for preparing gorgeous food for the guests and then eating out of a can, but I think sardines are beautiful, too! Plus, my body loves the protein and omega-3s. If you can't take the fishiness, look for a boneless, skinless variety in olive oil. You won't get AS MANY omega-3s, but you will still get them.

Total time: 20 minutes   **Yield:** 2 servings (2 fritters each)

1 tin sardines, drained

½ teaspoon minced garlic

2 green onions, finely minced

¼ cup (28 g) coconut flour

½ teaspoon baking powder

½ cup (30 g) fresh parsley, measured loosely packed and then finely chopped

1 egg

2 tablespoons (30 ml) avocado oil

Accessories needed:

Medium mixing bowl

Frying pan

Add the sardines, garlic, green onions, coconut flour, baking powder, and parsley to a medium mixing bowl and combine with a fork. Crack in the egg and mix until a thick paste/mixture comes together.

Heat the frying pan over medium-high heat and add the avocado oil. When it swirls easily around the pan, transfer the batter over in ¼-cup (60-ml) scoops. You can roll them into balls and slightly flatten for uniform-looking patties, or you can just drop and fry!

Fry for 2 to 3 minutes per side, until they are golden brown. Personally, I like dipping these in homemade tartar sauce whipped up from prepared mayonnaise, chopped gherkin pickles, a spoonful of capers, and a pinch of Old Bay Seasoning. Doing my omega-3 dance!

Nutritional Information: Calories: 355 – Protein: 20 g – Fat: 25 g – Carbs: 12 g – Fiber: 2.4 g – Net carbs: 9.6 g – Sodium: 341 mg – Potassium: 492 mg

Vegetarian Mains

Meatless Mondays—or any plant-based meal, for that matter—should be D E L I C I O U S! I love creating filling, balanced combinations that provide plenty of satiating fat and protein.

My friends and clients have gone positively mad for the completely vegan Macadamia-Ricotta Zucchini Lasagna Roll-Ups (page 164). And I love switching up Middle Eastern night with low-carb, protein-heavy Broccoli-Hemp Heart Falafel (page 170)! I recommend having those with the hummus, muhammara, and tzatziki from the Filling Snacks section—YUM!

Macadamia-Ricotta Zucchini Lasagna Roll-Ups

When I fed these roll-ups to my vegetarian bestie for the first time, she said, "this is my ultimate heaven!" and totally made my day. I've been making them for my meat-loving yet dairy-avoiding family, friends, and clients for ages, too. You really can't get any better than this easily portioned vegan lasagna with all of its good fats and assorted veggie goodness.

Total time: about 1 hour **Yield:** 4 servings (2 to 3 pieces each)

---

1 cup (240 ml) hot water

1 cup (135 g) macadamias (I used roasted and salted.)

1 pound (455 g) zucchini, cut lengthwise into ¼-inch (6 mm) strips

1 tablespoon (15 ml) extra-virgin olive oil

¼ teaspoon salt

⅛ teaspoon black pepper

⅛ teaspoon garlic powder

2 tablespoons (8 g) packed fresh basil

2 tablespoons (24 g) chopped tomato (1–2 grape or cherry tomatoes)

1 chopped green onion, white parts only

1 cup (240 ml) prepared low-sugar marinara sauce (I used Rao's.)

Accessories needed:

Baking tray

Parchment paper

Small bowl

Food processor or blender

Pie tin

Preheat the oven to 375°F (190°C, or gas mark 5). Line a baking tray with parchment.

In a small bowl, combine the hot water and macadamias. Set aside to soak. Lay out the thin strips of zucchini on the parchment. Brush each with the olive oil and season with the salt, pepper, and garlic powder. Bake for 18 minutes until pliable.

While these are baking, transfer the soaked macadamias with half of the soaking water into a food processor. Add the basil, tomatoes, and green onion. Blend until it has a ricotta consistency.

Once zucchini strips have been removed from the oven, line a pie tin with a piece of parchment paper and pour in ½ cup (120 ml) of the marinara sauce. On one end of each zucchini strip, add 2 tablespoons macadamia mixture. Roll toward the other end to form a tube and place with loose end downward in the sauce-lined pie plate. Repeat process until all zucchini is rolled up. Distribute remaining ½ cup (120 ml) of sauce on top of the roll-ups, and any remaining macadamia mixture on top and in between. Bake for 25 minutes. Remove from the oven and enjoy!

Nutritional Information: Calories: 350 – Protein: 5 g – Fat: 33 g – Carbs: 13.5 g – Fiber: 5 g – Net carbs: 8.5 g – Sodium: 470 mg – Potassium: 629 mg

Individual Eggplant-Tomato Stacks & Dairy-Free Basil Pesto

Eggplant Parmesan was the first recipe I remember helping my mother with when I was just knee-high to a grasshopper. Dredge-dip-dredge-and-fry. And our family barely ever actually got to eat eggplant Parmesan because we all stole the fried eggplant pieces before they could make it into a serving dish!

I decided I just *had* to "healthy up" one of my favorite childhood dishes, and this is it. We replace the usual breadcrumbs with LSA, a mixture of flax (linseed) meal, sunflower seeds, and almond flour, which you can buy premade in places such as Australia, but not yet in the United States.
So now you'll have a recipe for that, too!

Total time: 1 hour   **Yield:** 4 to 5 servings

LSA

½ cup (73 g) sunflower seed kernels

½ cup (52 g) almond flour

½ cup (63 g) golden flaxseed meal

Eggplant Stacks

1 cup (126 g) LSA

¼ teaspoon Italian seasoning

⅛ teaspoon salt

⅛ teaspoon pepper

1 pound (455 g) eggplant, peeled and sliced into ¼-inch (6 mm) slices

¼ cup (60 ml) extra-virgin olive oil, divided

4 Roma tomatoes cut into ¼-inch (6 mm) slices

4 ounces (115 g) fresh or shredded mozzarella

Dairy-Free Basil Pesto

1 cup (40 g) fresh basil

3 tablespoons (27 g) pine nuts

3 tablespoons (45 ml) extra-virgin olive oil

Accessories needed:

Blender or food processor

2 shallow bowls or pie tins

Baking trays

Parchment paper

Salt

Make the LSA: Combine all the ingredients in a blender and pulse until a smooth powder has been formed. Use to boost the nutrition of your salads and smoothies, AND as breadcrumbs like in this recipe!

Make the eggplant stacks: Preheat the oven to 400°F (200°C, or gas mark 6) and line baking trays with parchment paper.

Mix the LSA with Italian seasoning, salt, and pepper. Pour ¼ cup (about 32 g) into one bowl or pie pan and 2 tablespoons (30 ml) of the olive oil into another. Dredge the slices one by one in the olive oil and then coat with the LSA. Transfer to the baking tray and repeat process, including filling up bowls with additional oil and LSA, until all the eggplant is coated. Bake at 400°F (200°C) for 15 minutes, then flip and bake for 10 minutes.

Lay the slices of tomato on a parchment paper-lined tray and season with salt and pepper. Bake for 25 minutes, at the same time as the eggplant.

While they bake, make the pesto: Combine all of the ingredients in a blender or food processor and process until smooth. Season to taste with salt.

Once they come out of the oven, quickly build the eggplant into stacks of 4 slices with tomato and a sprinkle of mozzarella in between each eggplant piece. Pop back into the oven for 10 minutes to melt the cheese, then remove and enjoy with your pesto!

Nutritional Information: Calories: 544 – Protein: 13.1 g – Fat: 50 g – Carbs: 17 g – Fiber: 8.1 g – Net carbs: 8.9 g – Sodium: 800 mg – Potassium: 598 mg

Spinach-Lemon Pesto Zoodles with Half-Roasted Grape Tomatoes and Mozzarella

The zucchini noodles provide volume for this filling recipe, as well as a score of vitamins and minerals for minimal calories—our primary goal for eating nutrient-dense foods! You can make this a veggies on-veggies meal or use traditional spaghetti or another kind of noodle, if desired, though that will add to the total cooking time depending on package directions.

Total time: 40 minutes   **Yield:** 2 servings

½ cup (62 g) grape tomatoes, halved

Salt and black pepper

⅛ teaspoon garlic powder

2½ ounces (60 g) baby spinach

2 tablespoons (8 g) packed fresh basil

Zest and juice of 1 lemon

2 tablespoons (30 ml) extra-virgin olive oil, plus more if needed

2 tablespoons (18 g) pine nuts

1 small clove garlic

⅛ teaspoon salt

4 cups (480 g) zucchini noodles

4 ounces (115 g) bocconcini (fresh little mozzarella balls), torn in halves or quarters

Accessories needed:

Pie tin/small baking tray

Parchment paper

Blender or food processor

Medium mixing bowl

Preheat the oven to 425°F (220°C, or gas mark 6). Line a small baking tray or pie tin with parchment paper.

Place the tomatoes, cut-side up, onto tray. Season with salt, pepper, and garlic powder. Roast for 20 minutes.

While the tomatoes cook, place spinach, basil, lemon juice and zest, olive oil, pine nuts, garlic, and salt in a blender and blend until smooth.

Toss the zucchini noodles (which you can make at home with a spiralizer from a ¾ to 1 pound [340 to 455 g] zucchini OR purchase already made) with the pesto and taste. Adjust seasoning with additional salt and pepper.

By this time, the tomatoes should be ready to remove from the oven. Add them to the bowl of zoodles along with the torn bocconcini. Toss to combine. The heat from the tomatoes will slightly warm the zoodles and soften the mozzarella. Divide between 2 plates and enjoy!

Nutritional Information: Calories: 373 - Protein: 15 g - Fat: 30 g - Carbs: 14 g - Fiber: 3.6 g - Net carbs: 10.4 g - Sodium: 462 mg - Potassium: 912 mg

Broccoli-Hemp Heart Falafel

These glorious green falafels are almost effortless and are so well matched with Everyman Tzatziki (page 64), Sunflower Seed Muhammara (page 61), and the Low-Carb Spiced Cauliflower Hummus (page 62). Your body will love the ALA, protein, vitamins, and minerals from the healthy hemp hearts.

Total time: 30 minutes   **Yield:** 4 servings (about 4 pieces per serving)

2 cups (142 g) raw broccoli florets

½ cup (60 g) hemp hearts

1 tablespoon (7 g) ground cumin

½ tablespoon (6 g) ground coriander

½ tablespoon (9 g) Himalayan sea salt

½ teaspoon cayenne pepper

2 cloves garlic, minced

2 large eggs

3 tablespoons (21 g) coconut flour

¼ teaspoon salt

½ cup (33 g) packed fresh parsley

¼ cup (40 g) chopped onion

2 tablespoons (30 ml) extra-virgin olive oil

Accessories needed:

Food processor

Baking tray

Parchment paper

Nonstick or cast-iron frying pan

2-tablespoon (30 ml) portion scoop if handy

Line a baking tray with parchment. Combine all of the ingredients *except the olive oil* in the bowl of a food processor. Pulse to form a fairly smooth paste, stopping to scrape down the sides frequently.

Use a 2-tablespoon (30-ml) portion scoop, ⅛ cup measure, or tablespoon to measure out 2-tablespoon mounds. Place the mounds on the baking tray. There should be 15 to 16 mounds in the batch.

Once all are measured out, wet your hands slightly and roll each mound into a ball. Flatten slightly into a disc about ½ inch (1 cm) thick.

Heat a frying pan over medium heat until a drop of water sizzles on contact. Add ½ to 1 tablespoon (8 to 15 ml) of olive oil to the pan depending how large it is. If you can fit 4 pieces into the pan, use ½ tablespoon (8 ml). If you can fit 8, use 1 full tablespoon (15 ml).

Transfer the patties to the pan and cook for 1½ to 2 minutes per side, which should leave them with a crispy, golden edge. Transfer to a plate and repeat the process until all are cooked. Enjoy!

Nutritional Information: Calories: 266 – Protein: 13 g – Fat: 21 g Carbs: 11 g – Fiber: 3.4 g – Net carbs: 7.6 g – Sodium: 798 mg Potassium: 561 mg

Curry Vegetables with Dhal & Crunchy Almond Topping

This recipe is a little involved, but it's worth the time and effort. The delicious blend of spices and veggies provides so many anti-inflammatory nutrients while warming you up from the inside out.

Total time: 1 hour 10 minutes   **Yield:** 4 servings

Curry Roasted Vegetables

2 cups (226 g) cauliflower florets

1 cup (150 g) turnip in ½-inch (1 cm) dice

1 bunch rainbow chard separated into stems and leaves

½ cup (64 g) chopped red onion

2 tablespoons (30 ml) extra-virgin olive oil

½ teaspoon ground turmeric

½ teaspoon garam masala

¼ teaspoon salt

Red Lentil Dhal

1 tablespoon (15 ml) extra-virgin olive oil

½ cup (64 g) chopped red onion

1 tablespoon (10 g) minced garlic

1 tablespoon (6 g) minced fresh ginger

Salt

½ cup (62 g) chopped tomatoes

½ teaspoon garam masala

½ teaspoon turmeric

½ cup (96 g) dry red lentils

2 cups (475 ml) water

Crunchy Almond Topping

1 teaspoon coriander seeds

1 teaspoon cumin seeds

½ cup (70 g) chopped salted roasted almonds

1 finely chopped jalapeño (optional)

Accessories needed:

Baking tray

Parchment paper

Small saucepan

Pie tin

Preheat the oven to 375°F (190°C, or gas mark 5). Line a baking tray with parchment paper.

Make the vegetables: Place the cauliflower, turnip, chard stems, onion onto the baking tray. Drizzle with the olive oil and add the spices and salt. Toss well to coat all veggies. Bake for 30 minutes; then stir in chard leaves and bake for 10 minutes. Remove when done and set aside.

Make the dhal: While the vegetables cook, add the oil, onion, garlic, ginger, and a pinch salt to a small saucepan over medium-high heat. Sauté the garlic, onion, and ginger for 5 minutes. Add the tomatoes and spices and cook for 5 minutes. Pour in the lentils and cook for 2 minutes before adding the 2 cups (475 ml) of water. Bring to a boil. Cover and reduce the heat to low, allowing to simmer for 15 minutes, stirring occasionally. Remove from the heat and set aside.

Make the topping: Add the coriander and cumin seeds to a pie tin and roast at the same time as the vegetables, but only for 5 minutes! Remove, cool, and combine in a small bowl with almonds and jalapeño (if using).

To serve, place one-quarter of the dhal on a plate or in a bowl and top with one-quarter of the vegetables. Garnish with crunchy almond-seed-jalapeño mixture and enjoy!

Nutritional Information: Calories: 348 – Protein: 13.3 g – Fat: 20.5 g – Carbs: 33.3 g – Fiber: 9.1 g – Net carbs: 24.2 g – Sodium: 530 mg – Potassium: 992 mg

Sides

I just can't get enough veggies in my life, especially when they're this tasty! Vegetables in their whole spectrum of colors offer so many vitamins and minerals, to NOT add a stunning extra side dish to whatever you're eating would be a crying shame.

Double or triple the serving size and make Beet Noodles with Ricotta and Hazelnuts (page 178) a whole meal. Or make Amchoor Roasted Asparagus (page 162) as a perfect— and perfectly quick—side to the Bright Coriander Roasted Salmon (page 160).

Chili-Roasted Cauliflower Steaks

Did you know a pinch of chili flakes can boost both your metabolism *and* your mood? Capsaicin provides those benefits plus many more, and combined with superhero cauliflower, it's also flippin' delicious. Prepare yourself for just the right amount of heat while enjoying a delicious, healthy, cholesterol-lowering side dish.

Total time: 40 minutes   **Yield:** 4 servings

1 medium cauliflower (1½ pounds [680 g] or 5- to 6-inch [13- to 15-cm] diameter), cut into about six 1-inch (2.5 cm) steak-like pieces

2 tablespoons (30 ml) extra-virgin olive oil

½ teaspoon fine salt

¼ teaspoon crushed red pepper flakes

Freshly ground black pepper

Accessories needed:

Baking tray

Parchment paper

Preheat the oven to 400°F (200°C, or gas mark 6). Line a baking tray with parchment paper.

Drizzle each cauliflower piece with 1 teaspoon olive oil and rub all over. Sprinkle salt, crushed pepper flakes, and freshly ground pepper evenly over all pieces.

Place in oven and bake for 30 minutes. Remove and enjoy!

Nutritional Information: Calories: 97 – Protein: 2.8 g – Fat: 7.2 g – Carbs: 7.4 g – Fiber: 3 g – Net carbs: 4.4 g – Sodium: 335 mg – Potassium: 442 mg

Roasted Lemon Cauliflower Tabbouleh

Most cauli-tabbouleh recipes call for raw cauliflower, and although that can be tasty, it can also be a little harder to digest and not really emulate the texture of tabbouleh's normal bulgur. In this recipe, we give it a quick trip to Oven-town with lots of lemon zest, and it creates a whole new dish that is, in one word, phenomenal.

Total time: 35 minutes   **Yield:** 4 servings

2 cups (226 g) cauliflower rice

2 tablespoons (30 ml) extra-virgin olive oil, divided

¼ teaspoon salt, plus more to taste

Finely grated zest of 1 lemon

1 cup (135 g) peeled and small-diced cucumber

½ cup (62 g) small diced tomatoes (I like to use cherry or grape tomatoes—more lycopene, too!)

1 green onion, chopped finely

Juice of 1 lemon

1 bunch fresh parsley, leaves only

Accessories needed:

Baking tray

Parchment paper

Medium mixing bowl

Preheat the oven to 400°F (200°C, or gas mark 6). Line a baking tray with parchment paper.

Spread the cauliflower rice on the baking tray and add 1 tablespoon (15 ml) of olive oil, salt, and lemon zest. Combine well and spread into a thin layer across the tray. Pop into the oven for 20 minutes.

Meanwhile, in the mixing bowl, combine the cucumber, tomatoes, green onion, lemon juice, and remaining oil. Set aside.

Once the cauliflower comes out of the oven, allow to cool for at least 5 minutes before adding to the mixing bowl so you don't "cook" the raw vegetables. Fold it and the parsley in at the same time. Chill it in the fridge for 10 minutes before you dig in!

Nutritional Information: Calories: 91 – Protein: 1.8 g – Fat: 7.1 g – Carbs: 7.4 g – Fiber: 2.6 g – Net carbs: 4.8 g – Sodium: 77 mg – Potassium: 309 mg

Wild Mushroom Cauliflower Risotto

This low-carbohydrate risotto is rich, thanks to the cream and cream cheese, and oh-so-comforting. Plus, it provides health-promoting phytochemicals from the mushrooms and cauliflower.

Total time: 30 minutes   **Yield:** 2 to 4 servings

6 ounces (168 g) assorted wild mushrooms, sliced

2 tablespoons (30 ml) extra-virgin olive oil, divided

⅛ teaspoon salt

⅛ teaspoon black pepper

⅓ cup (55 g) minced onion

3 cups (340 g) cauliflower rice

½ cup (120 ml) water

¼ cup (60 ml) heavy cream

2 tablespoons (30 g) cream cheese

Chopped fresh herbs (optional)

Accessories needed:

Baking tray

Parchment paper

Large frying pan

Preheat the oven to 400°F (200°C, or gas mark 6). Line a baking tray with parchment paper.

Place the sliced mushrooms on the baking tray and drizzle with 1 tablespoon (15 ml) of olive oil, salt and pepper. Toss well to make sure there's no mushroom left behind and spread in a single layer on the tray before putting in the oven. Bake for 15 minutes, until the mushrooms are starting to get golden.

While they cook, add remaining tablespoon olive oil to the frying pan. Add the onion, cauliflower rice, and a pinch more of salt. Sauté, stirring frequently, for 8 minutes when the onion and cauliflower will be starting to get a little soft. Add the water and allow it to steam through. When the water has almost completely evaporated, lower the heat to medium and stir in the cream and cream cheese.

By the time the cream cheese has melted, the mushrooms should be out of the oven. Pour them directly into the frying pan and combine with the creamy cauliflower rice. Remove from the heat and garnish with chopped fresh herbs (if using)! Parsley goes great here and boosts the nutrition even more!

Nutritional Information (based on 3 servings): Calories: 227 – Protein: 4.3 g – Fat: 20 g – Carbs: 11 g – Fiber: 3.8 g – Net carbs: 7.2 g – Sodium: 66 mg – Potassium: 469 mg

Beet Noodles with Ricotta and Hazelnuts

Sweet beets, creamy ricotta, crunchy toasted hazelnuts, and a fistful of baby spinach make for one nutritious and ultra-textured meal. You can use washed and thinly sliced beet greens instead of baby spinach if you buy them in a bunch and want to avoid food waste.

Total time: 25 minutes   **Yield:** 4 servings

1 pound (455 g) raw beets, any color

2 tablespoons (30 ml) extra-virgin olive oil

1 tablespoon (15 ml) apple cider vinegar

2 green onions, chopped finely

Salt and black pepper

½ cup (67 g) hazelnuts, chopped

2 cups (60 g) baby spinach

8 ounces (225 g) ricotta cheese

Balsamic reduction (optional)

Accessories needed:

Baking tray

Parchment paper

Spiralizer

Medium mixing bowl

Pie tin

Preheat the oven to 400°F (200°C, or gas mark 6). Line the baking tray with parchment paper.

Peel and spiralize the beets. Place in mixing bowl with olive oil, vinegar, green onion, and a pinch of salt and pepper. Toss well to combine and transfer to the baking tray. You may need to trim noodles so they're not too long.

Place in the oven and bake for 10 minutes. While they are baking, put the hazelnuts in the pie tin. Once the 10 minutes has passed, put the nuts in the oven to toast and leave the beets in there for 5 minutes.

Remove the nuts and beet noodles from the oven at the same time and *immediately* stir the baby spinach through the beet noodles to wilt it slightly.

Spread the ricotta on a serving plate in a thick layer. Top with the beet noodles and wilted spinach, and garnish with the toasted nuts! Season to taste with salt and pepper. Drizzle on a little balsamic reduction if you want to further sweeten it up!

Nutritional Information: Calories: 286 – Protein: 11 g – Fat: 20 g – Carbs: 17 g – Fiber: 5.1 g – Net carbs: 11.9 g – Sodium: 158 mg – Potassium: 655 mg

Ras el Hanout Roasted Red Cabbage

This cabbage gives people the same joy that bacon does. There, I said it. For one vegetable, a plate of this has about four different textures and even more flavor notes. This pairs really well with the Easy Antioxidant Pumpkin Tagine (page 91) and the Bright Coriander Roasted Salmon (page 160), but don't take my word for it. Try some of this purple deliciousness yourself!

Total time: 1 hour 10 minutes   **Yield:** 6 servings (1 wedge per serving)

1 pound (455 g) red cabbage (You can substitute green if you must, but you will lose those particular purple veggie health benefits!)

2 tablespoons (30 ml) extra-virgin olive oil

½ tablespoon (4 g) ras el hanout spice blend

1 teaspoon Himalayan salt

Accessories needed:

Baking tray

Parchment paper

Preheat the oven to 350°F (175°C, or gas mark 4). Line a baking tray with parchment paper.

Cut cabbage into wedges that are about 1 inch (2.5 cm) at their thickest on the outside of the wedge. Lay them on the baking tray. Drizzle with olive oil, sprinkle with ras el hanout and salt. Toss lightly and rub the pieces together to ensure that they all get coated with both oil and seasonings.

Place the tray in the oven and bake for 30 minutes, until the edges of the cabbage are nice and golden brown. After 30 minutes, remove the tray from the oven and cover with foil before popping back in for 30 minutes. Now it will steam and get all tender in the closed packet.

Remove after 30 minutes, serve, and enjoy!

Nutritional Information: Calories: 60 – Protein: 1 g – Fat: 4.6 g – Carbs: 4.6 g – Fiber: 2 g – Net carbs: 2.6 g – Sodium: 338 mg – Potassium: 132 mg

Broccolini With Buckwheat and Ricotta Salata

Buckwheat is a flavorful pseudo-cereal (meaning a seed that is consumed as a grain but does not grow on grasses). It has an impressive micronutrient profile, hearty flavor, and low effect on blood sugar due to its fiber content. When combined with superfood broccolini, bright lemon, a pinch of spice, and a little creamy salty cheese, you get a multi-textured, complex-flavored dish with incredible nutrition.

Total time: 30 minutes   **Yield:** 4 servings

1 bunch broccolini or 1 stalk regular broccoli cut into 1-inch (2.5 cm) pieces

2 tablespoons (30 ml) plus ½ teaspoon extra-virgin olive oil, divided

Freshly ground black pepper

Pinch crushed red pepper flakes

1 cup (240 ml) water

¼ teaspoon salt

½ cup (82 g) kasha (toasted buckwheat)

2 ounces (55 g) crumbled ricotta salata (Feta will work, too.)

Zest and juice of 1 lemon

Accessories needed:

Baking tray

Parchment paper

Medium saucepot with a lid

Serving bowl

Preheat the oven to 425°F (220°C, or gas mark 6). Line a baking tray with parchment paper.

Spread the broccolini out in a single layer. Drizzle with 1 tablespoon (15 ml) of oil and sprinkle with salt, freshly ground black pepper, and crushed red pepper flakes. Bake for 15 to 20 minutes until it is easily pierced with a fork and lightly browning.

Boil water with salt. Add the kasha and bring back to boil. Cover and turn heat to low for 10 minutes, setting timer. Once the timer goes off, remove from the heat and uncover.

Once the broccolini comes out of the oven, transfer the kasha to a mixing or serving bowl, add broccolini, ricotta salata, lemon zest and juice, and remaining olive oil. Combine and season to taste with additional salt and pepper.

Nutritional Information: Calories: 193 – Protein: 6.1 g – Fat: 11 g – Carbs: 19 g – Fiber: 3.1 g – Net carbs: 15.9 g – Sodium: 267 mg – Potassium: 216 mg

Amchoor Roasted Asparagus

Amchoor powder is a tart, bright spice made from pulverized dried green mangoes traditionally used in India. It is PACKED with nutrients, including vitamins A, C, E, antioxidants and iron. You can find it at many grocery stores in the spice section and also Indian markets.

Prep time: 30 Minutes **Yield:** 4 servings

1 pound (455 g) fresh asparagus

2 tablespoons (30 ml) extra-virgin olive oil

¼–½ teaspoon salt

Freshly ground black pepper

½ teaspoon amchoor powder

Accessories needed:

Baking tray

Parchment paper

Preheat the oven to 400°F (200°C, or gas mark 6). Line the baking tray with parchment paper.

Break the tough ends off of the asparagus and peel if the stems are thick. Place them on the baking tray in a single layer and drizzle with olive oil. Sprinkle with salt, pepper, and amchoor powder. Toss in the tray to make sure all pieces are well-coated.

Bake for 25 minutes, until the tips start to brown and the stems are crisp-tender. Enjoy!

Nutritional Information: Calories: 84 – Protein: 2.5 g – Fat: 6.9 g – Carbs: 4.8 g – Fiber: 2.4 g – Net carbs: 2.4 g – Sodium: 267 mg – Potassium: 233 mg

Best Garlic-Roasted Broccoli

This might just be the simplest roasted broccoli recipe you ever come across. It has tons of texture and flavor, as well as a good amount of healthy inflammation-reducing monounsaturated fat!

Prep time: 35 Minutes **Yield:** 4 generous servings

1 pound (455 g) broccoli, broken into bite-sized florets

¼ cup (60 ml) extra-virgin olive oil

½ teaspoon fine salt

½ teaspoon garlic powder

Accessories needed:

Baking tray

Parchment paper

Preheat the oven to 400°F (200°C, or gas mark 6). Line a baking tray with parchment paper.

Add the bite-sized florets to the baking tray. Drizzle with olive oil, salt, and garlic powder and toss well to coat. Place in the oven and bake for 30 minutes.

Nutritional Information: Calories: 159 – Protein: 3.2 g – Fat: 14 g – Carbs: 7.8 g – Fiber: 3 g – Net carbs: 4.8 g – Sodium: 328 mg – Potassium: 363 mg

Balsamic Vegetable Julienne

This dish is fast—so fast—and so tasty. You may just fall in love with celeriac, the more formal name for the mildly flavored celery root, after this. Considering that it contributes to strong and healthy bones, has an incredible macronutrient profile, and supports healthy digestion and immune function, that love affair would be a wonderful thing.

Prep time: 15 Minutes   **Yield:** 4 servings

1 celeriac bulb (about 1 pound [455 g])

1 cup (110 g) julienned carrot

½ cup (58 g) thinly sliced onion

½ cup (75 g) julienned red pepper

1 tablespoon (15 ml) extra-virgin olive oil

2 tablespoons (30 ml) balsamic vinegar

Salt and black pepper

Accessories needed:

Mandoline with julienne attachment OR julienne peeler

Medium mixing bowl

Large frying pan

Pare away the tough outer skin of the celeriac/celery root. Julienne with your tool of choice. Combine the vegetables in the mixing bowl and mix well, pulling apart any bits that didn't quite separate.

Heat the olive oil in a large frying pan over medium-high heat until it flows easily. Add the vegetables and a pinch of salt. Sauté until the vegetables are getting soft and pliable. Add the balsamic vinegar and toss the veggies while it steams through. Once the liquid is evaporated, it's done! Adjust seasoning with salt and pepper.

Nutritional Information: Calories: 109 - Protein: 2.4 g - Fat: 3.9 g - Carbs: 17 g - Fiber: 3.5 g - Net carbs: 13.5 g - Sodium: 137 mg - Potassium: 506 mg

Roasted Brussels Sprouts with Umami Caramel

You haven't lived until you've tasted these sweet, salty, umami Brussels sprouts! Making them takes two kinds of cooking, but it's worth it in the end, I promise.

Total time: 45 minutes   **Yield:** 4 servings

4 cups (352 g) cleaned and quartered Brussels sprouts

¼ cup (60 ml) coconut aminos or fish sauce

2 tablespoons (30 ml) water

2 tablespoons (18 g) erythritol, granulated monk fruit, or coconut sugar

Accessories needed:

Baking tray

Parchment paper

Steamer (or just a bowl and some plastic wrap to use in the microwave)

Small saucepan

Preheat the oven to 425°F (220°C, or gas mark 6). Line a baking tray with parchment paper.

Using a steamer of any type (bamboo, metal, in a saucepan, over a frying pan), steam the trimmed sprouts for 10 minutes until they can be lightly punctured with a fork but are not soft. While they are steaming, combine the aminos, water, and sugar/sugar substitute in the small saucepan over medium-high heat. Bring to a quick boil while whisking constantly to dissolve the sweetener as much as you can. Remove from the heat after 3 to 5 minutes and set aside to cool.

Once the steaming is done, transfer the sprouts to the baking tray and pour over the sauce. Toss the sprouts so that all are coated and transfer baking tray to oven. Roast for 25 minutes, until they start to brown. Remove from the oven and just try to eat one serving!

Nutritional Information: Calories: : 73 – Protein: 3 g – Fat: 0.3 g – Carbs: 17 g – Fiber: 3 g – Net carbs: 13.7 g – Sodium: 290 mg – Potassium: 343 mg

Recommended Reading

The Complete Guide to Fasting: Heal Your Body
Through Intermittent, Alternate-Day, and Extended Fasting
by Jason Fung, M.D., and Jimmy Moore

The Obesity Code: Unlocking the Secrets of Weight Loss
by Jason Fung, M.D.

Delay, Don't Deny: Living an Intermittent Fasting Lifestyle
by Gin Stephens

Useful Apps

Fasting

Zero
zerofasting.com

LIFE Fasting Tracker
lifeapps.io/apps/life-fasting-tracker

Meditation

Insight Timer
insighttimer.com

Headspace
headspace.com

Calm
calm.com

Meal Planning

PlateJoy
platejoy.com

Pepperplate
pepperplate.com

Plan to Eat
plantoeat.com

Ends+Stems
endsandstems.com

Yummly
yummly.com

About the Author

CHEF NICOLE POIRIER is an accomplished special-diets chef with 20+ years of experience facilitating nutritional healing through delicious, mindful eating. Always on the leading edge of culinary wellness trends, she founded Mind Body Keto in 2017 to advocate a holistic approach to the on-trend ketogenic diet, incorporating her passion for the health benefits afforded by intermittent fasting in 2018.

Nicole began writing about increasing wellness through tailored nutrition as far back as 2011, though promoting it with her clients came long before that! She has a unique respect for the myriad dietary requirements people face and believes that the vast majority of health challenges can be overcome with the application of proper, nutrient-dense, whole food based eating. She shares keto, paleo, and more low-carb, special diet, and allergen-friendly recipes on her website mindbodyketo.com and Instagram account, @mind_body_keto.

Acknowledgments

Wow—writing a cookbook is such a wild, demanding, and fulfilling endeavor! I am so grateful for all of the hands that held mine, cheered me on, and pushed me forward during the process. To Tasha Metcalf, the most rad chick ever for connecting me to the opportunity; to Quarto/Fairwinds for believing that I had it in me; to Jill, Jenna, Renae, Heather, Cara, Todd, and all who have touched and edited and encouraged throughout—my cantankerous self couldn't have done it without you; to Gin Stephens & Dr. Jason Fung for providing the inspiration to find this amazing path; to Cedar, Harmony, the Honey Hive, Bec, Tiffany, and Gabé for celebrating with me from the get-go; to amazing friends and fellow authors Ariane Resnick and Simone Miller who helped me navigate this whole process; to every amazing love-note-sender when I was under the gun; and finally, to every reader, fan, and follower—my dream is for YOU, too, to find greater health and happiness with every bite.

Index